HOW TO SURVIVE YOUR HOSPITAL STAY

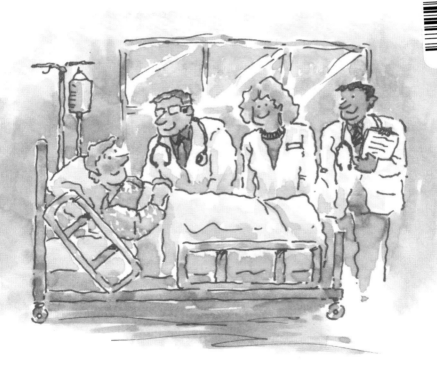

JUDY BURGER CRANE, RN

ILLUSTRATIONS BY JASON YOUNG

THE CENTER PRESS

Library of Congress Cataloging -in- Publication Data

Crane, Judy Burger, 1930-
    How to survive your hospital stay / Judy Burger Crane:
        Illustrations by Jason Young.
        ISBN 1-889198-02-1   p. cm.
        1. Hospital patients. 2. Hospital care. 3. Consumer education.
        Includes biographical references and index.
I. Title.
   RA965.6.C72   1997
   363.1'1- - DC21   97-26727
                            CIP

ISBN 1-889198-05-6 for plastic binding

Published by
        The Center Press
        30961 W. Agoura Rd. Suite 223-B
        Westlake Village, CA 91631
        (818) 889-7071 FAX (818) 889-7072

Cover design: by Bart Design Associates
Book design: by Bart Design Associates
Printed in USA.

10 9 8 7 6 5 4 3 2 1

TABLE OF CONTENTS

ABOUT THE AUTHOR   i

ACKNOWLEDGEMENT   ii

DISCLAIMER   iii

READERS GUIDE   v

1. GOOD NEWS, BAD NEWS   1
   What is contained in the Patient's Bill of Rights
   and how it pertains to you. How to be a better
   health care consumer. How to use this book.

2. CHOICES   3
   How to find the best hospitals and how to
   interview and choose the best doctors for
   you. Do HMO patients have any choices?

3. QUESTIONS, QUESTIONNAIRES AND
   OTHER PAPERWORK   9
   How can you prepare ahead of time for all
   those questions you will be asked? What
   questions should you ask? How to get
   reasonable answers to all your questions.

4. WHAT IF?   15
   What do you need to know concerning legal
   documents such as consent forms? How do
   you arrange for someone else to make medical
   decisions for you if you are not able to do so?
   Should the worst happen, do you want to
   donate organs to benefit others?

5. THE BOTTOM LINE - WHO PAYS?   19
   Understanding different types of health
   insurance and choosing the best one for
   your needs. What questions should you ask
   before choosing a new plan? What are your
   options if you don't have health insurance?

6. COUNTDOWN 25
What can you do to prepare for your
hospital stay? Things you'll be glad you
brought with you and things you'll wish
you had left at home.

7. 5:00 A.M.? YOU'VE GOT TO BE KIDDING! 33
What is the admitting process and why does
it take so long? What are the procedures that
will prepare you for surgery?

8. HOW'S THAT? 35
Navigating your way through the medical
maze of Latin words, abbreviated terms
and acronyms commonly heard on a
medical-surgical unit.

9. THE DESIGNER GOWN AND OTHER INDIGNITIES 39
"Why do I have to wear this dreary garment
with the built-in air-conditioning right where
I don't want it?", plus answers to questions of
a more personal nature.

10. THIS WON'T HURT A BIT 43
What should you know about pain shots,
IVs and blood drawing? What should you
do if you are a needle chicken?

11. WAKING UP IS NOT HARD TO DO 47
What are the different types of sedation?
Communicating with your anesthesiologist
while you are awake.

12. WHO ARE ALL THESE PEOPLE? 53
The patient's guide to Who's Who in the
hospital. Educational backgrounds and job
descriptions of RNs, LVNs, Nursing Assistants,
Residents and other hospital personnel.

13. HELLO, OUT THERE   61
   What is your nurse doing out there while
   you lie in the hospital bed? A sample morning
   in the life of your nurse.

14. WHO'S IN CHARGE?   65
   Nurses, doctors, patients - who is responsible
   for what and how you can do your part.

15. VISITORS - GUIDELINES   71
   Visitors - how to spruce up your hospital
   etiquette. What if you don't want to bring
   flowers? Here are some novel gift ideas
   that patients really appreciate.

16. DOUBLE OCCUPANCY   77
   How to get along with your roommate. What
   can you do about a difficult roommate situation?
   Helpful suggestions for maintaining your privacy.

17. CHILDREN, BABIES AND HOSPITALS   81
   How can you prepare your child for hospitalization? How can you prepare a child for a parent's
   hospitalization? What are your options if you
   are a breastfeeding mother and must be
   hospitalized? Information for expectant parents.

18. HOW DO I GET OUT OF THIS PLACE?   87
   Why should you plan ahead for your discharge
   from the hospital? What can you do if you think
   your discharge is premature?

19. HOW CAN I EVER THANK YOU? OR SHOULD I?   93
   Showing appreciation for the care you received
   is a nice way to complete your stay. On the
   other hand, how can you voice your complaints
   effectively and who should you talk to?

20. HOME, SWEET HOME   97
     Why it is important to get back into your
     routine gradually. Five important lifestyle
     changes you can make. What support is
     there for people with chronic medical
     conditions? How to use your doctor or
     the Internet to find the support group
     that best meets your needs.

     PATIENT'S BILL OF RIGHTS   101

     REFERENCES AND RESOURCES   107

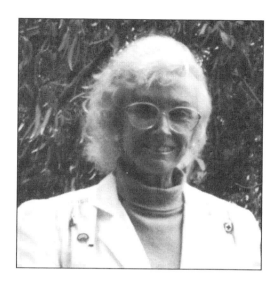

ABOUT THE AUTHOR

Judy Burger Crane has been a medical-surgical nurse for twenty three years, first at UCLA Medical Center, then at Santa Monica-UCLA Hospital. Her experiences have included staff nursing, managing nursing teams, and designing and teaching classes for nurses.

Patient education is a vital part of an RN's job. Helping patients and families to understand their medical problems, and teaching them how to cope once they are discharged from the hospital, is very important. Judy finds a great deal of satisfaction in this part of her work. In writing *How to Survive Your Hospital Stay*, she hopes to educate prospective hospital patients, their families and friends about how the system works, what their rights are, and how to obtain the care that they need in order to have the best possible recovery.

In addition to her experiences in hospital nursing, she is a volunteer with the American Red Cross. She also does volunteer work in the Community with children.

ACKNOWLEDGEMENTS

I wish to thank Bernard Selling, writer, gifted teacher, and friend for his confidence in my ability to write this book and his "nudging" me to get on with it.

I am indebted to my fellow writers and friends for their honest critiques and encouragement - Selma and Arnold Patent, Tobie and Arnie Robinson, Diane Hanson, Maygene and Fred Giari, and Fran Wofford.

For their professional point of view and input, a special thanks to Diana Faulk, CRNA; Randall Parker, MD; Helen Parker, Patient Ombudsman; Leslie M. Eber, MD, FACC; Scott Bateman, MD; and Cheryl Uelmen, RN.

My favorite patient, Beryl Hart, contributed a unique bedside point of view. Her ideas sparked two important chapters: "Hello Out There" and "Double Occupancy."

For their technical expertise and artistic contributions, I am grateful to Mar Puatu, Jason Young, and Rene and Jim Moore.

My family have been wonderful in their contribution of ideas and ongoing support. Thanks to my Aunt Virginia, Christine, Shawn, Andy, Leslie, Howard, Michele and Mark.

The love and confidence of my husband, Elie, and my mother, Marjorie, have encouraged and inspired me to write this book.

WARNING - DISCLAIMER

The author has designed this book to provide information and suggestions in regard to the subject matter covered. It is sold with the understanding that the publisher and author are not engaged in rendering medical, legal or other professional services. If medical or other expert assistance is required, the services of a competent professional should be sought.

This book is not intended to reprint all the information that is otherwise available to the patient/prospective patient, but to encourage the seeking of information suitable to the individual's needs.

Every effort has been made to make this book as accurate as possible. However, there may be typographical errors. Additionally, different hospitals, insurance systems and medical personnel may operate in ways different from that described in this book. This book should be used as a general guide, not as the ultimate source of medical information.

The purpose of this book is to educate. The author and publisher shall have neither liability nor responsibility to any person or entity with respect to any loss or damage caused, or alleged to be caused, directly or indirectly, by the information or suggestions contained in this book.

If you do not wish to be bound by the above, you may return this book to the publisher for a full refund.

READER'S GUIDE

Diabetes, out of control.
Kidney failure.
Bowel obstruction.
Pneumonia.
Congestive heart failure.
Stroke.

These are just a few of the many ailments that put people in the hospital. Hospitalization is the last resort when a medical problem cannot be taken care of in the doctor's office or at home. Sometimes a hospital stay is anticipated, such as for a hip replacement. At other times, however, it comes as an unpleasant surprise. Accidents or sudden onset of an illness can result in Emergency Room visits and subsequent hospitalization. In another scenario, your doctor might decide that an illness has worsened and needs treatment in the hospital.

"I'm sorry to tell you," your doctor announces after listening to your lungs during an office visit, *"your congestion is worse and I'm afraid you have pneumonia. I'm going to admit you to the hospital."*

The good news is that if you need surgery, there is a possibility that it will be done as an outpatient procedure.

The management of medical problems has changed greatly in the last ten years and still is changing at a rapid rate. Many surgical procedures have been refined so that they are less invasive and are performed in a shorter time. Patients spend less time under anesthesia and often go home the same day.

Outpatient Departments have grown and are used for many surgeries as well as non-surgical procedures such as chemotherapy and tests which require some form of sedation.

However, whenever it is necessary to be admitted to the hospital, either unexpectedly or as a planned event, much of what takes place does not have to be news to you, the patient.

Throughout this book, an attempt is made to address medical as well as surgical situations. All but two of the chapters are relevant for both. Chapter Seven outlines the admitting procedures for a surgery patient. Chapter Eleven describes both General Anesthesia, which might be used for major surgeries, and Monitored Anesthesia Care, which might be used for a breast biopsy, for example. All of the other chapters, however, describe situations that pertain to medical, surgical or obstetrical patients, alike.

No matter what the reason is for hospitalization, it is important for you to know that you not only have a right to ask questions, but that it is vital for you to do so. You also have a right to reasonable answers and explanations.

This book emphasizes the patient's role in the management of his health care as it guides patients and families from the begining to the end of a hospital stay. Read it and make full use of the **NOTES** pages to record your questions, the answers you receive, as well as any concerns you have throughout your stay.

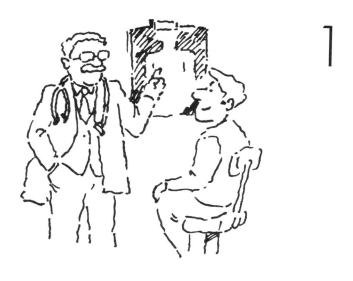

1

GOOD NEWS,
BAD NEWS

"Well, I have good news and I have bad news," your family doctor tells you, peering over his glasses. *"The bad news is that you have a blockage in your colon."*

Your heart sinks. *"That's terrible,"* you say. *"Quick, tell me the good news."*

He smiles. *"The good news is that we can remove the blockage by performing surgery in the hospital, and you won't have those pains in your abdomen anymore."*

"Hospital?" you shout. *"I hate hospitals! Can't you just give me some pills?"*

You don't think the good news is all that wonderful, do you? Well, you're not alone. Being admitted to a hospital is not high on the 'fun' list for most of us. You've heard horror stories about how Aunt Minnie got pneumonia in the hospital, about surgeons removing the wrong leg, and hospital bills in tens of thousands of dollars. On the other hand, if the problem is "fixable" that is good news.

This book takes you step-by-step from the time the family doctor announces that hospitalization is necessary (either for surgery or for a medical problem) all the way to discharge with prescriptions and instructions in hand. You will find checklists for use in discussions with physicians, tips on what to pack and what to leave at home, as well as a list of frequently used medical terms.

In this book you will find explanations for the procedures you will go through, from admission to discharge. Included are descriptions of the different professional licensed and other trained personnel you will encounter, and many tips for getting through a hospital stay with the least amount of anxiety.

Nurse's Notes are scattered throughout the book. These are first-person anecdotes from a nurse's experiences on a medical-surgical unit. Some are funny, some are poignant, and all are true.

There is more good news. As a patient you have choices and it is important that you make educated choices. Your choices will be educated if you know your rights — the right to ask questions and the right to be given reasonable answers. In the Appendix you will find a copy of *A Patient's Bill of Rights*. It is important that you read and understand this document published by the American Hospital Association.

To be a better informed patient read this book before your admission to the hospital, and take it with you to review different chapters, as necessary, during your stay. Use the **NOTES** page at the end of most chapters to make lists of questions to ask the doctors or nurses and to write down the answers, or just to write information you want to remember later. This will help you to be a more informed patient.

You may be surprised at how smoothly everything will go when you understand what you can expect and what is expected of you.

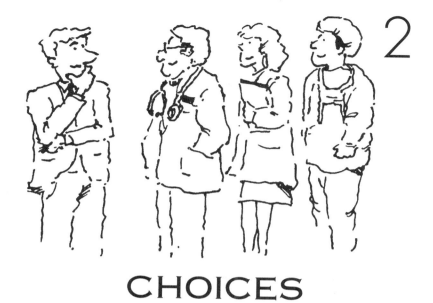

CHOICES

"How do I choose a surgeon?" you ask your primary care doctor. He has recommended surgery and wants you to be evaluated by a surgeon.

"I recommend Dr. Johnson," your doctor replies. *"He is excellent and has performed many of these surgeries."*

You trust your doctor's judgment, but still you hesitate. Is Dr. Johnson really the one for you?

Well, guess what? You don't have to decide right this moment (unless your problem is of an urgent nature). You have choices. *"I appreciate your recommendation,"* you tell your doctor. *"I'd like to make some inquiries on my own. If I come up with different recommendations, I'll run them by you."* A reasonable doctor will not object. If you undergo surgery your physician wants you to be comfortable that you made the right choices.

How does one choose a surgeon or specialist, and for that matter, how does one choose a primary care doctor?

Nurse's Notes	*"I'm having surgery next week," my neighbor tells me. "Dr. Jones is going to fix my foot problem." "Good," I reply. "How did you happen to choose him?" "Oh, my cousin says he's wonderful," she answers. "He goes to her church. She says he's very friendly and active in Little League!"*

For a start, ask your friends and family for their recommendations. Have they had a similar medical or surgical problem? Was there good follow-up? What did they like and not like about a particular physician? Check with your insurance representative and physician referral services which are available at some hospitals. As you narrow your choices, consider proximity to your home.

When you're shopping for furniture or a new car, you do some research, taking into consideration your needs and your lifestyle. Picking a primary care doctor, a surgeon or other specialist, deserves at least as much attention.

Before agreeing to any procedure, do some reading about your medical problem and the possible solutions. The more you know, the better questions you can ask. Libraries and the Internet are good resources.

Remember, you as the patient play an important part in making these choices. The more you know and communicate, the better your care and recovery will be.

O.K. You've done your homework. You're ready to *interview* the top names on your list of primary care doctors. Make appointments. Organize your medical history and bring any pertinent records with you such as results from MRI, CAT scans, angiograms, stress tests, etc. State at the outset of each interview that you are looking for a new primary care doctor.

Ask the doctors about hospital affiliations. Find out who is on-call in their absence and whether or not the on-call physician has access to your records. How do you feel in your conversation with the doctors? Do they listen to you? Do they acknowledge your feelings and concerns? Do they give you reasonable answers, or do they dismiss your questions as uninformed or unimportant? You want to establish a relationship with a primary care physician (either an internist or a family practice doctor) you can trust. Never have surgery without discussing it thoroughly with your personal physician.

When meeting for the first time with a surgeon or specialist, ask yourself the same questions. Do you feel confident and comfortable with him or her? In addition, ask about board certification (i.e., the completion of an accredited residency and the passing of an exam given by a specialty board). Is the surgeon specialized in the type of surgery you need? How many of these operations has he or she done? You may have other questions. Add them on the **NOTES** page.

Feel free to tell your primary care doctor that you want a second or even a third opinion, especially if this is major surgery, e.g., a hysterectomy. Keep in mind that not all insurance will pay for a second opinion. If you do go to another doctor, take all your test results, and X-rays with you.

After your meetings with the new physicians, go home and talk it over with your family or a friend. Then make your decision. Yes, this person is qualified, or I want to look further. If you narrow it down to two equally competent physicians, choose the one with a smile and an optimistic disposition. You, after all, are the consumer. YOU HAVE CHOICES.

You also want to check out the hospital. Find out if it is accredited by the Joint Commission on Accreditation of Healthcare Organizations (write to JCAHO, One Renaissance Blvd., Oak Brook Terrace, IL 60181, or call (708) 916-5600). How often does the hospital deal with your specific condition? Is it routine in that facility or a rarity?

Does the hospital have a house staff, i.e., physicians on duty at the hospital 24 hours a day? In other words, if you develop a serious problem in the middle of the night, is there an in-house doctor who can come to see you right away? Or do they have to call a doctor at home to come in?

If you are having sugery, and your local hospital is limited as to the types of surgeries routinely performed or does not have a house staff, you may want to ask your primary physician to refer you to a larger hospital where your particular type of surgery is done more often and where there is a house staff of competent physicians.

You can play an important role in maximizing your chances for a good outcome by educating yourself and asserting your rights. By doing this, you will know that you are making good choices.

NOTES

NOTES

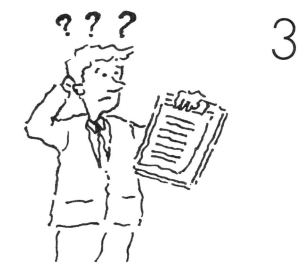

3

QUESTIONS, QUESTIONNAIRES AND OTHER PAPERWORK

"Do you have any allergies?"
"Any history of diabetes in your family?"

Your family doctor has referred you to a surgeon or specialist. You are in his office, waiting your turn and filling out a questionnaire on a clipboard. The family doctor has all this information. You wonder why you have to answer all these questions again. It will seem like everyone you encounter in the medical system is asking you the same questions. Don't these people ever talk to each other?

9

It's called documentation. Each office you visit, each system you enter has its own set of records. Yes, your family doctor has your medical history right up to last week. Now, the specialist you are about to meet needs to make out his own records. He will want to hear from you what you are allergic to, what previous surgeries you might have had, and what medications you are currently taking.

In addition, the Admissions Office at the hospital will have questions for you, and a nurse on the floor where you are admitted will have many questions - most of which you have already explained to the surgeon. In each place, the physicians, the hospital, and the nurses must keep their own records. They each have a professional as well as a legal responsibility for their part in your care. You have a responsibility too. It is to provide the health care personnel with accurate information about yourself so that they can do their jobs.

Abdominal surgery is used here as an example. However, the information on how to traverse the path from home to doctor's office to hospital and back home is basically the same no matter what the surgery or medical procedure.

Now, the paperwork. You can do it the hard way or the easy way. Either way you are going to do it. Paperwork is as inevitable as sunrise.

The hard way:

You can sit there in the waiting room racking your brain trying to remember when you had that hernia surgery, how old your father was when he died, and what's the name of that blood pressure medication you're taking. OR —

The easy way:

You've read this book. You have taken five minutes at home before coming to the surgeon's office, and you have made a list (a 3 x 5 card is handy) of the following information which you will be asked on the questionnaire or by the surgeon in person:

- What are your symptoms? What makes it worse; what makes it better? Be sure to include signs which may not seem relevant to you, but may give the doctor important additional information, e.g., weight changes, increase in thirst, frequency of urination.

- Is there a family history of this particular problem? Are your parents living? If not, at what age did they die, and of what cause? Siblings - same questions.

- What prescription medications are you taking? Name, dosage, how many per day? How about over-the-counter drugs, e.g. aspirin or Tylenol, antacids? Cough medicine? Laxatives? Every day, or just occasionally?

- Are you exposed to unusual chemicals or substances at work? Is your job particularly stressful?

- Are you allergic to any medications? Any foods? Anything that goes on your skin, like soap? If you have had an allergic reaction, what form did it take? Rash, swelling, difficulty breathing?

- Have you traveled out of the country in the last six months?

- Have you had recent contact with anyone who has developed an illness?

- The last question the surgeon will probably ask you is, "Do you have any questions?"

It's finally your turn!

Yes, you have a few. Last night at about 3:00 a.m. you had several hundred running through your head. "Am I going to die?" was only one of the many horrible possibilities you were mulling around.

This is broad daylight, however, and you are prepared. You have made out a list of questions and now go over it with the physician who will be directing your care. Here are some of the basics. Tailor them to fit your particular situation, and add questions of your own on the **NOTES** page at the end of this chapter.

1   Is there an alternative therapy to this surgery?
2.   Does it have to be done now, or can it wait until
        a. My insurance kicks in?
        b. After my vacation?
        c. I finish final exams in two weeks?
        d. My baby is older?
        e. My mother-in-law leaves? Arrives?
3.   Can you draw me a picture of where the problem is and where the incision will be?
4.   Will there be a scar?
5.   Will I be asleep during the surgery?
6.   What are the risks? Are there any aftereffects?
7.   How painful will it be? What will be done to alleviate the pain?
8.   How long will I be in the hospital? If I want some one to stay overnight with me in the hospital, how do I arrange that?
9.   When can I go back to work? Drive a car?
10.   Will this surgery affect my sexual activity?
11.   Should I stop taking my medications before the surgery? Should I bring my medications to the hospital? Will the nurses be giving me the same medications?
12.   Will I need a blood transfusion? Can I donate my own blood ahead of time (autologous blood)?
13.   What can I do to best prepare myself for surgery?
14.   Will I need physical therapy or a visiting nurse when I go home? Who arranges that?

Remember, *YOU ARE THE CLIENT.*

The doctor is the provider of a service. You have a right to ask any question and to receive a reasonable answer. When it comes to your own body, no question is dumb and no subject too personal to discuss with your doctor. Most doctors will answer your questions intelligently. They want you to be well-informed. Ask your question once, and then listen carefully to the response. Then write down the answers you get.

Look at the following hypothetical conversation between a patient and a surgeon.

> *Patient:* "Will I be asleep during surgery? I'm worried about the anesthesia."
>
> *Doctor:* "Now don't you worry about that. Just let me take care of everything."

This is not a reasonable answer. Our patient isn't going to be put off so easily.

> *Patient:* "I would like you to tell me what kind of anesthesia will be used and what its effects will be. I want to write that down."
>
> *Doctor:* "We will use a general anesthetic. You will be asleep during the whole procedure."

That's a reasonable response. If you want more details, you can ask.

It's your body. You have a right to know what's going to happen to it.

If your attempts at communication with the specialist leave you uneasy, call your family doctor and discuss it with him. Perhaps he can answer your questions. If you are still dissatisfied, perhaps you will decide to interview another specialist on your list.

YOU HAVE CHOICES!

13

NOTES

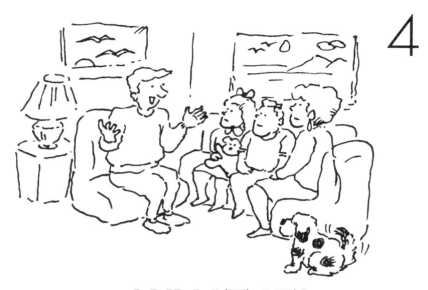

4

WHAT IF?

You know what "What Ifs" are. They are the pesky little thoughts that creep in through the back door of your mind and keep you awake in the wee hours.

> *"What if I change my mind after I sign the consent for the procedure?"*
> *"What if I'm brought into a hospital too sick to speak up for myself?"*
> *"What if this procedure doesn't resolve the problem?"*

You are going to have questions and concerns, but you can significantly reduce the number of "What Ifs" by educating yourself ahead of time.

Informed Consent

Prior to any surgery or invasive procedure, whether in the hospital, doctor's office or clinic, you will be asked to sign an informed consent. Yes, more paperwork. This is a very important piece of paper. Read it carefully. Informed consent means the patient, guardian or surrogate decision-maker was made aware of the risks, benefits, and alternatives to the proposed procedure and then gave his or her permission to proceed. If you still don't understand some aspect of the procedure, now is the time to ask.

"Tell me again, Doctor. What are the up-sides and the down-sides to this surgery?"

The consent will state the name of the procedure, which side will be operated on (e.g., left leg, right thumb) and the name of the doctor performing the procedure. You will be given a copy of the consent.

"What if I change my mind after I have signed the consent?"

You have the right to change your mind about a procedure at any time. If this occurs, the issue will be resolved between you and your physician. However, the likelihood of you having a change of heart is less if you have educated yourself about the potential procedure.

There are two legal issues you should know about before you are admitted to a hospital. In fact, these should be considered before you are ill or need surgery.

Advance Directive

Every adult has the right to accept or refuse any recommended medical treatment. For most of us, it is hard to imagine ever being too weak or so distracted by pain and anxiety as to not be able to speak for ourselves. For the most part, hospital patients are awake and alert and able to make these decisions for themselves.

Unfortunately, during severe illness people are sometimes unconscious or otherwise unable to communicate their wishes. In that case, the Advance Directive would help your doctors and family make decisions that are in your best interests and follow your wishes.

In the Advance Directive (in some states called Durable Power of Attorney for Health Care Decisions) you state your wishes regarding various medical treatments, and you appoint someone (a family member or close friend) to make medical decisions for you if you are unable to do so. This person knows your feelings and wishes about such issues as blood transfusions, as well as extreme life-saving measures such as kidney dialysis, artificial ventilation, etc.

Advance Directive forms are not the same in every state, though use of your home state's legal forms usually assures acceptance in another state. Ask your physician how to obtain a copy. Stationery stores that carry business and legal forms might have them in stock. (See the Resources section for other sources.)

Every adult should consider having an Advance Directive. Make sure your physician and members of your family have copies of yours. Don't put it off. Do it now. While you're ordering your form get extras for other members of your family. You may be the one making the decisions for them some day. Find out now what their wishes are.

Organ Donation

It is difficult for most of us to really accept the fact that one day we will leave this world. When that time comes, your family may be faced with the question, *"Are you willing to donate your loved one's heart or kidney so that another human being might live?"*

This is an incredibly difficult decision for a family to be asked to make at the height of their grief. The most loving thing you can do is to make your wishes known now, in writing on your Advance Directive and in discussions with your family. Let them know whether you do want your organs made available, or that you do not want them to make an organ donation. Or tell them they can make that decision when the time comes.

Including your organ donation wishes in your will isn't effective. By the time your will is read, donation will not be possible. Carrying an Organ Donor card in your wallet is a good idea.

In any case, for now you can make certain decisions while you are hale and hearty. Take care of as many of those "What Ifs" as possible before the need arises.

NOTES

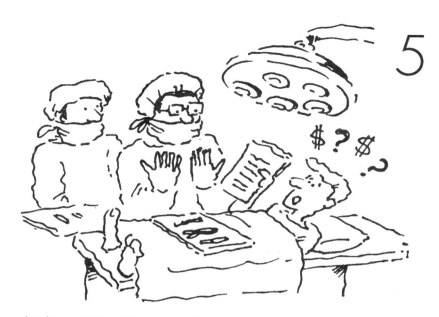

THE BOTTOM LINE - WHO PAYS

Don't read this chapter if you have medical insurance, you're happy with it, and are confident that you understand as much about it as you care to. Health insurance is complex, confusing and continually changing. It also makes for dry reading. You could save this chapter to read some night when you're having trouble falling asleep. If you choose to read on, however, don't say you weren't warned!

"How much is this going to cost me?"

That's one of the questions you were worried about at 3:00 a.m. If you must spend any time at all in a hospital, it is important for your peace of mind, to know in advance who pays what to whom.

19

If you are one of those fortunate enough to have health insurance, your insurance company (the primary payor) will pay all or a portion of your medical bills and you will pay a co-pay or the balance. If you have a supplemental policy (secondary payor), it will pay all or most of the balance. To eliminate unpleasant surprises, it is important to know whether your doctor is a provider for your particular plan.

The two main categories of health insurance are Indemnity/Fee for Service and Managed Care Plans.

Indemnity/Fee for Service

In this type of health insurance you pay a premium, either individually or through your employer, to an insurance company. You may go to any doctor or hospital and the insurance company will pay a portion - usually 80% - of reasonable and customary medical costs. You or the supplemental policy are responsible for the balance. These plans sometimes do not cover preventive care.

If you are covered under two policies (a husband's employer and a wife's employer, for example) your own insurance (the primary) will cover the major portion of the costs with the spouse's policy (the secondary) picking up all or most of the balance.

Managed Care

Managed care is an umbrella term which includes several types of plans that closely supervise care and restrict patients' choices of doctors in order to control costs. These include health maintenance organizations (HMOs), point-of-service (POS) plans and preferred provider organizations (PPOs).

HMOs charge premiums to the individual or the employer and provide health care for a small co-pay fee from the patient and rarely charge for necessary hospital stays. Usually, claim forms are not required and care must be coordinated through a primary care physician whom you choose when you join the plan from the network of doctors belonging to that particular HMO.

Primary care doctors are usually family practice physicians, internists, obstetrician/gynecologists, or pediatricians. It is the primary care doctor, often described as a gatekeeper, who provides, arranges, or authorizes all of your care. You need a referral from your primary care physician and approval from the HMO before visiting any medical specialist. You may go to a hospital only with the advance approval of the primary care doctor and the HMO, except in emergencies. In any HMO the quality of care depends largely on the physician group and the efficiency of the referral system.

The POS plan allows members to receive care either in or outside of a network. Out-of-network care usually costs more and requires members to pay up front and then file claim forms to be reimbursed.

Who pays if you have Medicare and elect to join an HMO? The HMO has an agreement with the U.S. Government, whereby the HMO administers the health care benefits of Medicare recipients who decide to join. In return, the Government pays the HMO a fixed monthly amount for each person served. There are no deductibles or paperwork, and the individual is limited to the providers and the procedures of the HMO.

The PPO option is a plan in which a group of doctors, hospitals and other providers agree to provide health care services at negotiated rates. In this plan, the patient chooses providers as the medical need arises (physicians, optometrists, dentists, etc.) from a list. These "preferred providers" agree to accept a set fee for their services from the insurance company, and there may or may not be a balance to be paid by the patient.

The structure of healthcare delivery is changing. Health insurance coverage is complicated. This is by no means a complete description. You need to find out in advance what kind of plan you have, what is covered and what is not. You need to know what your deductibles are and when they apply. When making an appointment with a doctor or a laboratory, or contemplating a hospital stay, inquire whether or not they accept your insurance.

If you are in the process of choosing a new health care plan, here are some issues to consider:

- Is your own doctor on the plan's list?

- If not, can you choose your new doctor? Will you see that doctor each time?

- Is the doctor's office in a convenient location?

- Do you have a choice of hospitals?

- What do you do in case of an emergency? Where do you go? Who decides if your problem is an emergency?

- Are you covered for any existing medical conditions?

- If you are a woman, can you see a gynecologist for routine gynecological services, or must you see your primary care physician for those services? Does the plan cover a mammogram and pap smear every 1-2 years?

- If you are a man, does the plan cover a test for prostate cancer (PSA) every year?

- What appeal process for treatment decisions does the plan have in place?

- Does your plan pay for a second opinion?

- What is the procedure for changing primary care doctors if you are not happy with the first one you chose?

READ THAT LAST QUESTION AGAIN.

The major theme of this book is that YOU HAVE CHOICES. No, you will not be struck by lightning if you decide that you are not compatible with the first or even second physician you pick. Hey, it's your life, your body, your health.

YOU ARE A CLIENT, NOT A CAPTIVE.

❦❦❦

Most people are healthy when they enroll in a health care plan and may select a plan primarily on the basis of its cost. Its real value is determined by the quality of the care it provides when you are ill. Choose well.

❦❦❦

What if you don't have insurance coverage? Ask your doctor if you can set up a payment schedule. Inquire at the hospital in advance how you can arrange payments. Perhaps this surgery or procedure could be scheduled for a later date. Or maybe you qualify for treatment in a clinic where your fee would be based on your income.

It is important for your recovery that you not have these worries hanging over your head, so do your homework.

NOTES

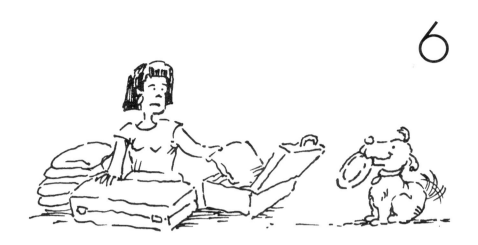

COUNTDOWN

H-Day, Minus Seven

"Poor Fido! Who's going to cater to your every whim while I'm in the hospital?"

This, and other chores need to be arranged for in advance. Don't leave everything until the last minute.

A week or more before your anticipated hospital stay prepare your house and your household for your absence. If you live alone, do some of the following:

1. Find a pet-loving friend to care for Fido or Calico. Leave them with plenty of food (don't forget the can opener) and the name, address and phone number of the veterinarian as well as the location of the pet carrier box.

2. Stop the newspaper and have the Post Office hold your mail, or arrange for a friend or neighbor to pick up your paper and mail.

25

3.   See if this kind person will also water your plants.

Whether or not you live alone include some of the following on your H-Day, Minus Seven List:

4.   Pay in advance any bills that may come due or arrange for a later payment.

5.   Mail birthday cards and gifts for occasions that will occur in the next week or two.

6.   Look in your closet for a bathrobe that you aren't ashamed to be seen in.

7.   If you have children, confirm your child care arrangements.

8.   If you are breastfeeding, see Chapter 15.

9.   Arrange for a friend or family member to take you to the hospital and bring you home. It is preferable that the person bringing you home isn't someone who has to do it on a lunch break. Discharge procedures sometimes take longer than anticipated.

10.   Start practicing some relaxation exercises.   Sit quietly in a chair. Close your eyes. Do some deep, slow breathing. Breathe in through the nose and out through the mouth. Relax your muscles—one part of your body at a time. Visual imagery can be helpful. Imagine a peaceful spot and picture yourself enjoying its quiet solitude. See the References and Resources section for some good reading and listening on relaxation techniques. Do them each day before going into the hospital and use them for maintaining a healthy mental attitude while you're there.

11. You may want to notify your minister, priest, or rabbi. Spiritual support can be very helpful during an illness.

12. You may want to visit the hospital in advance of your day of admission. Ask at the front desk if you may visit the floor where surgery patients go after surgery.

Locate the Nurses' Station and introduce yourself.

"Hi, my name is Mary Wells. I'm having surgery next week and I guess I'll end up on this unit. Is it possible for me to meet the Charge Nurse?"

Ask directions to the Surgery Waiting Room where your family members or friend can wait during your surgery. If you have been instructed to come to the hospital several days in advance of your admission to be pre-admitted this is a good day to do your familiarization tour.

H-Day. Minus Two

Take it or leave it? Today is the day to pack, so what do you take and what do you leave at home? For starters, picture your hospital room. You will have a bed. There will be a bedside stand with one drawer that you can reach if you bend your wrist just right unless you have an IV in that hand. There will be a cupboard below that you couldn't open from a lying position even if you could reach it, which you can't! You and your roommate will share a cupboard the size of a broom closet for your clothes.

Following are two lists. Tailor them to your own needs and the anticipated length of your hospital stay.

TAKE IT

- Eyeglasses.
- Cheap watch, only if you can't stand not to know what time it is.
- Phone numbers of friends & family.
- Your 3 x 5 card (see Chapter 3).
- List of medications you are currently taking, including dosages, e.g., Accupril 20 mg, once a day.
- Health Insurance, Medicare, or Medicaid card.
- Aforementioned bathrobe.
- Slippers with sturdy, non-skid soles.
- Toiletries - toothbrush & tooth paste, denture cup and cleansing tablets, comb or brush, deodorant.
- Shaving equipment - disposable or battery-operated razors only. Hospital safety regulations prohibit the use of personal electrical devices.
- Cosmetics - Visitors expect you to look pale and wan. You don't need a vanity case full of stuff. But take whatever will make you feel good.
- Clothes to wear home, keeping in mind where you might have an incision. Sweat suits or jogging suits are good.
- Change of underwear and socks (NOTE: Bring colored socks and underwear. White articles of clothing can get scooped up with the sheets and tossed in the laundry.)
- Copy of your Advance Directive.
- Paperback book, magazines to catch up on. Don't try to read *War and Peace* in the hospital. It's (a) too long, (b) too heavy to hold when you're reclining in bed, and (c) takes more concentration than you probably will have.
- Eye mask and ear plugs. Hospitals are bright and noisy places.
- Note pad and pen, to make note of questions to ask your doctor on his daily visit.

LEAVE IT

- Cares and Woes. Do what you can about problems at home and at work, and try not to worry about what you can't do.
- Perfume. You might find your favorite fragrance downright sickening as you come out of the anesthetic. Also, your roommate might not appreciate it.
- Wallet, credit cards.
- Electrical appliances - anything that plugs in. Hospital safety regulations prohibit personal electrical equipment. (Battery-operated is OK)
- Money, the possible exception being some change for newspapers or taxi fare if you will be taking a cab home.
- Jewelry.

Nurse's Notes	
	My new patient is about 60 years old and has a long scraggly beard. *"Did you bring anything of value?"* *I ask him.* *"No," he responds. "Well, yes, there's just my little gold nugget. And my gold cross. I'm a miner."* *My mouth drops open. I try to maintain my professional composure.* *"Could I see the nugget, please?" I ask. "I've never seen one before."* *He pulls out his handkerchief and unwraps it. his "Little" gold nugget is the size of a golf ball!* *"Why did you bring it with you?" I ask.* *"I was afraid someone might steal it from my trailer," is his calm reply.* *P.S. We put his nugget and cross in the hospital safe.*

H-Day. Minus One

"Nurse, I haven't had a bowel movement in four days. Could you please call my doctor for a laxative?"
Don't let this be you. It's a delicate subject, but an important bodily function. Try to arrange your diet so that you have normal movements during the few days before hospitalization. Do a mental check on this today.

If you are a smoker, it's a good idea to stop before and for as long after surgery as possible. A study out of Houston's Baylor College of Medicine says smokers who quit smoking - even temporarily - heal faster from wounds and surgery. Many hospitals do not permit smoking except in certain outdoor areas, so be prepared to do without. (This would be an ideal time to consider quitting.)

"I'll just have this teensy half cup of coffee before leaving for the hospital in the morning." No. Don't do it!

If you are having surgery or tests, you will be given instructions about when you may have your last food and/or drink. There are reasons for the rules. Follow them. In any case, you would be wise to eat lightly the day before entering the hospital for surgery or tests.

You're all set. Try to have a relaxing evening, and get to bed early. You have to be at the hospital at 5:00 a.m.

NOTES

NOTES

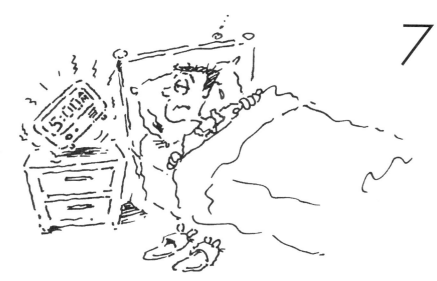

7

5:00 AM?
YOU'VE GOT TO
BE KIDDING!

"Why do I have to be there at 5:00? My surgery isn't until 9:00." That's a reasonable question. The answer is that you have several stops to make before you show up in the operating room.

The first stop is Admitting (unless you have been pre-admitted several days before). Here you are officially admitted to the hospital and your records are put into the computer. You will be asked to sign a hospital admission agreement. Be sure to bring with you your Social Security number, your medical insurance card(s) or Medicare and Medicare supplement cards, and the name, address and phone number of the person to contact in case of emergency. This can be family, next of kin, or a close friend.

As soon as you arrive on the floor where you will be admitted, your nurse will have forms to fill out. Here's where you are asked some of the same questions you were asked by your doctors: Allergies? Medications? History of illnesses, surgeries? (Aren't you glad you brought your list and your 3 x 5 card?) Nurses have their own responsibilities for your care, and will start a chart which will follow you throughout your hospital stay.

The surgeon's orders will have preceded you, and the nurse has already made sure that the appropriate medications are on hand.

Arriving on time gives everyone plenty of time to do their job. If your surgeon has ordered a pre-operative medication, the extra time allows it to take effect, whether it is an antibiotic or something to relax you. It also provides for some quiet time before you go to the operating room.

So lie back, do some deep breathing and relaxation exercises and put yourself in capable professional hands.

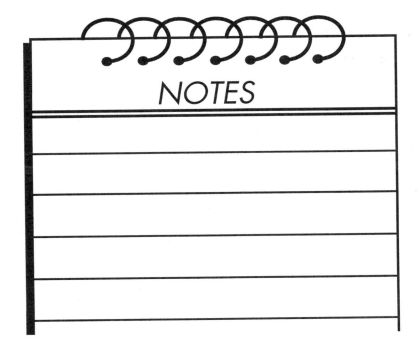

NOTES

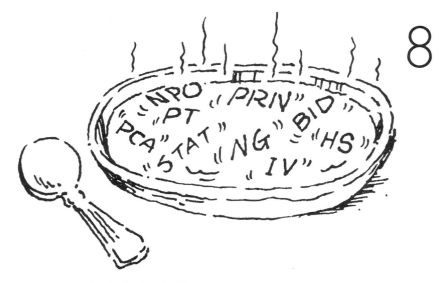

8

HOW'S THAT?

"*Hi, Mr. Freedman, I'm Susie, your Pre-Op RN,*" says Miss Chipper. "*I'll be starting your IV, and giving you a pre-op med. You'll be glad to know that your EKG and CBC results came back normal. Have you been NPO since midnight?*"

You're who? You're going to do what? Have I been what?

Say what? You're in Hospital Country now, so be sure to bring with you this guide to Medicalese. Some of what Susie Chipper, RN just said to you makes sense. Let's translate the whole thing.

Susie has just informed you that she is a licensed Registered Nurse (RN), and is in charge of you during this pre-operative period. She will insert an intravenous line (IV), or catheter, into a vein in your arm. This line is connected to a plastic bag of fluid, usually dextrose (sugar) or saline (salt) or a combination. The fluid will keep you from becoming dehydrated since you are not able to drink. This line is also used to give you medicines intravenously.

She is further explaining that before you leave for the operating room, she will give you an injection of a medication to relax you. Your Complete Blood Count (CBC), shows a normal number of red and white blood cells, and your Electrocardiogram (EKG), shows your heart rhythm to be normal. She is asking if you have been NPO (Latin for non per os), meaning refrained from food or drink, since midnight.

Following is a list of terms you may hear and equipment you may encounter during your hospital stay. Don't let it scare you. Not all of it will pertain to you.

NG Tube - Nasogastric tube - a tube placed through the nose and down into the stomach. Used either to keep the stomach empty or for liquid feedings when a patient is unable to swallow.

Catheter - a tube:
Urinary (Foley) catheter - placed through the urethra into the bladder to drain urine.
Cardiac catheter - passed into the heart through a vein or artery.

Void - to urinate (as in "Have you voided yet?").

Stool - bowel movement (as in "Was there any blood in your stool?").

Emesis - vomit (as in "When you threw up, what color was the emesis?").

Vital signs - BP - Blood Pressure
Temp - Temperature
Pulse
Respirations

Aqua pad/K pad - a heating pad with pre-set temperature.

Analgesic - pain relieving medicine.

PCA - Patient Controlled Analgesia - a narcotic syringe connected to the IV line. When the patient has pain, he pushes a button and a small, regulated dose of pain medication is administered through the IV. The amount of medication per dose and the number of possible doses per hour is prescribed by the doctor. The machine is then pre-set according to those orders. It is not possible for the patient to receive too much medication.

TED hose/Antiembolic stockings - very tight stockings, knee-high or thigh-high, to promote good blood circulation and prevent swelling.

Pneumatic Boots - boots (though they don't look like boots) that are wrapped around the legs. The boots inflate with air and then deflate. This continues as long as the machine is turned on. They serve the same purpose as TED hose.

NPO - refrain from food or drink.

Meds - medications:

Routine - every day at specific times:

  qd - every day

  BID - twice a day

  TID - three times a day

  QID - four times a day

  hs - bedtime (hour of sleep)

PRN - as needed, pain medication, e.g.

po - by mouth.

IM - intramuscularly

IV - intravenously (through the IV)

Labs - laboratory test results.

I & O - Intake and Output - a record of all fluids taken in, both IV and oral, and all fluids out, including urine, emesis and anything out of an NG tube.

Practice some of these terms ahead of time. The natives may look at you with new respect.

"Oh Nurse, I drank this cup of juice. Do you want to put it on my I&O sheet?"

"Are you going to give that medication IV or IM?"

On the other hand, when medical personnel approach you with words and phrases unfamiliar to you, don't hesitate to ask for clarification.

Lab tech: "Hi, Mr. Freedman, I'm Ted. I'm here to draw a.m. labs for renal lytes."

Patient: "Hi Ted. I don't know what renal lytes are. Could you please explain that?"

Lab Tech: "It's a blood test to check your glucose level and your kidney functioning."

It doesn't have to be a secret language to you. You may have already picked up a good bit of medical terminology from watching television. Now's your chance to really understand what they're talking about. Write down some of the terms you hear on TV and ask your nurse what they mean. You can be the family interpreter.

NOTES

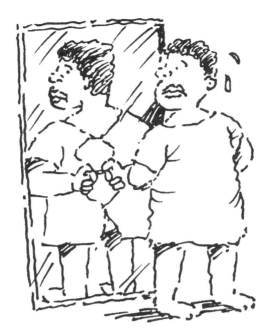

9

THE DESIGNER GOWN, AND OTHER INDIGNITIES

"Take all your clothes off and put this gown on," Nurse Chipper tells you. *"It ties in the back."* You look in dismay at the shapeless garment.

You follow her instructions, undressing in the privacy of your curtained-off bed. Now you check yourself in the mirror. The gown is white with a little blue design. If you are 6'2" and weigh 250 lbs., the gown hits you about mid-thigh. You check out your backside in the mirror and are appalled to see said backside in full view where the gown doesn't come together. If you are 5'2" and weigh about 110 lbs., it will be plenty long and wrap around you twice.

Across the front, stamped prominently in black, are the words "PROPERTY OF WE CARE HOSPITAL, DO NOT REMOVE." Well, there goes your plan of sneaking a few of them home with you to give as Christmas presents!

Other indignities include questions of a personal nature which you will be asked by the nurse.

"When was your last bowel movement?"
(You were ready for this one - you read
   Chapter Six last week.)
"Do you drink alcohol? How much? Several
beers a day? One cocktail a week?"
"Do you use any other substances, e.g.
recreational drugs?"

This could be important for the nurses and doctors to know in the event that you will be receiving anesthesia and/or pain-relievers containing narcotics. This is not intended to lecture you about your lifestyle. Hospital personnel are solely concerned with your medical needs and the possible interaction of different drugs.

Are these indignities necessary? The information about your personal habits, like smoking or drinking, could be very important as you progress through your hospital stay. Nurses and doctors need to assess you each day. The more they know about what you put into your body, the better they are able to take care of you. Whether or not it's good for you is your responsibility.

On the other hand, if you do not wish to answer a particular question, you have the right to say, "I decline to answer."

And the designer gown? Is there a reason for this snappy design? It certainly brings new meaning to the word *generic*. On the plus side, the gown makes it easier for the doctor to examine you and for the dressings to be changed. Also it doesn't bind up as pajamas would when you turn in the narrow bed.

Helpful hint: As you are recovering from your illness or surgery, and are able to walk to the bathroom or in the hall, ask your nurse for an extra gown to put on the other way, tied in front. That should cover everything.

NOTES

NOTES

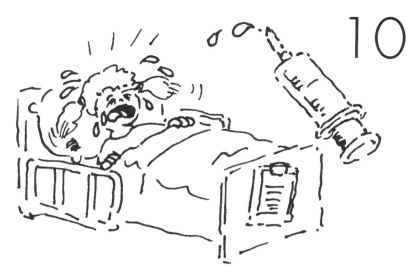

THIS WON'T
HURT A BIT

"Just a little needle stick. Hold real still now." WHAM!
"There, that wasn't so bad, was it?"

No, your arm is just throbbing and feels like a balloon. You take a tentative peek at the arm. Well, it looks pretty normal, but it sure hurts. The nurse has put a needle into a vein in your arm and is busy connecting some plastic tubing to it.

"What's all this?" you ask.

"Oh, just some IV fluids your doctor ordered," she answers.

You, however, have been doing your homework. "What are the fluids, and what will they do for me?" you ask.

"This is dextrose and saline," she responds. *"Since you are NPO (Nothing by mouth - see Chapter 8) this will keep you well hydrated."*

There are three different procedures requiring needle punctures through your skin which you will possibly encounter while in the hospital.

Intravenous Infusion (IVs)

The first is an IV, or intravenous. The IV catheter is a very small plastic tube with a needle inside which just protrudes from the catheter. The needle is used to enter a vein, usually in the hand or arm. Then the plastic catheter is threaded into the vein and the needle is withdrawn. The catheter is connected to a plastic bag via plastic tubing. This bag contains a liter (approximately a quart) of fluid, usually dextrose, normal saline, or both.

The IV gives you a measurable amount of fluid, and provides a way of administering medications, like antibiotics. During a period of time when you are not allowed any liquid or food, this keeps you from becoming dehydrated. Your doctor orders the amount and type of fluid and the medications, so it varies, but the procedure for inserting an IV is the same. If you need a blood transfusion, this line can also be used for that purpose.

Take a minute to look at the veins in your hand and arm. Whether they are prominent or are hard to see, the persons inserting the IV or drawing the blood know where your veins are located. We're all built pretty much alike.

However, veins are as individual as people when it comes to being prodded. Some scoot to one side when the needle is pushed against them - called rolling. Some, especially in older patients, are very fragile, and blow or tear when they are punctured by the needle. This is as distressing to the nurse or technician as it is to the patient, but, of course, it is the patient who has to suffer another needle stick.

If the nurse or technician has difficulty, and has to make two or three attempts, it's OK to ask for a break.

A responsible nurse will stop after three tries and

ask someone else to take over, perhaps a nurse from another department who is known to be able to get even the tiniest or most elusive of veins. A real professional will not consider it a loss of face to ask another nurse to try.

Sometimes a vein does not react kindly to having a plastic catheter inserted and left there for several days. Understandably. What does the vein know or care about your medical problems? If the site where your IV has been inserted becomes red or swollen or painful, immediately notify the nurse in charge of your care. Your IV will have to be moved to a different site, another vein, probably on the other arm. The redness, swelling, or pain will subside.

Blood Drawing

Uh oh! Here comes Dracula from the laboratory. He wants a sample of your blood for the lab tests. This is another procedure requiring a needle into your vein. Whatever the reason for your being in the hospital, it is likely that you will have blood drawn. It is usually taken from a large vein on the inside of your elbow. Blood drawing is done by a licensed technician (phlebotomist) or an RN.

Pain Medication

The pain shot comes as a mixed blessing . It may hurt going in, but gives you relief from the pain you are having as a result of surgery or your medical problem. This injection of pain medication, or analgesic, is most often given into a muscle in the buttock, though it can be administered in the thigh or the upper arm.

Other methods of receiving pain medication don't involve shots. One is epidural where a catheter is inserted during surgery into the epidural space that surrounds the outer covering of the spinal cord. Analgesics are administered into the catheter by the anesthesiologist who assesses the patient's level of pain relief each day.

Another is Patient Controlled Analgesia (PCA). A narcotic syringe is connected to the IV. When you feel pain, you push a button and a small premeasured dose is administered into your IV. If you push the button too often, it's OK. The regulator won't let you receive more than the allotted dose. If you are not getting good pain control, you tell the doctor or nurse, and the dosage can be adjusted.

Whether you are having an IV started, having blood drawn or receiving a pain shot, it is important to let your nurse know if needle sticks are particularly traumatizing for you. Ask the nurse to use all the tricks possible for making it easy on you.

"Just a little stick" is a medical euphemism for, *"Most of my patients say it does hurt, but I want to minimize your fear so you'll be relaxed."* There are people who have a very high pain threshhold, i.e. a high tolerance of pain. These individuals, indeed, barely flinch when getting immunizations or receiving pain shots. Others are truly traumatized by the mere sight of a needle. Then there is everyone else in between.

Wherever you are on the spectrum, it's OK. There's no good or bad, no babies or heroes. That's just you.

Let the person doing the needle sticking know which of the following is you:

A. *"Please explain what you are going to do before you do it. I like to be forewarned."*
B. *"Just do what you have to do, and let me know when you're finished so I can unclench my teeth and open my eyes."*
C. *"Shots don't bother me. Don't worry about it."*

Communication is the key word. You want to be comfortable, and the nurses want you to be as comfortable and pain-free as possible. So when someone comes at you with a needle, speak up.

11

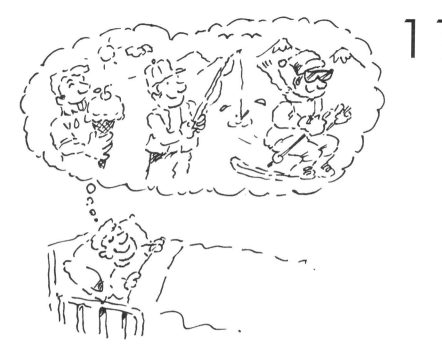

WAKING UP IS NOT HARD TO DO

Going Into and Coming Out of Anesthesia

"What if I don't wake up?"

It's only human to worry about handing control of our consciousness over to someone else. If this is a concern of yours, you are not alone. The person responsible will be either: an **anesthesiologist** – a physician who has specialized in anesthesia, or an **anesthetist** – someone medically trained to administer anesthesia, for example, a CRNA (Certified Registered Nurse Anesthetist). The term, anesthesiologist, will be used here. However, hospital practices differ, and either might be assigned to work with your surgeon.

47

Ask your surgeon which it will be and when you will be able to meet with and talk to this person. However, in most cases the anesthesiologist is chosen by the surgeon or is scheduled on a rotating basis by the hospital. They often utilize the hospital as their base of operations and do not have a separate office.

The usual procedure is that the anesthesiologist visits you in your room the night before surgery if you are, in fact, hospitalized prior to the day of surgery. If you are admitted on the morning of surgery, the visit will take place before you go into the operating room — perhaps in a pre-op holding area. You will be asked questions about your allergies and about previous anesthesia experiences. Take this opportunity to express your concerns and ask your questions.

"I'm really nervous about being put to sleep."
"Will I be able to feel any pain?"
*"The last time I had surgery, I was so
nauseated afterwards."*
"I want to be awake." "I don't want to be awake."

The anesthesia which is used to make you comfortable and pain-free during surgery, may be a General, a Regional or Local, or Monitored Anesthesia Care (MAC). The choice will depend on the area of the body to be operated on, the extent of the surgery, your medical condition, and your feelings about it. The type of anesthesia can be adjusted to keep you most comfortable.

It is definitely OK to ask questions and discuss your preferences with the anesthesiologist. Jot them down ahead of time on the NOTES page. If you are the kind of person who likes to know all the details you can write the answers there too.

Types of Anesthesia

General - Designed to inhibit nerve impulses to the operative site, and to induce amnesia and muscle relaxation. The patient is unaware of stimuli or surroundings. Oxygen is administered and a sedative is given through the IV to make the patient unconscious. Then the anesthesia is administered via a tube inserted through the mouth, down into the lungs, or by a mask over the mouth and nose, or through the intravenous line.

Regional or Local - Used for surgery on a small area of the body. Local anesthesia blocks nerve impulses without causing unconsciousness. Novacaine is a localizing agent used for numbing areas of the jaw prior to dental work. With regional anesthesia a larger area, such as an arm or a leg, is desensitized with localizing agents. Regional anesthesia includes epidural and spinal anesthesia.

Monitored Anesthesia Care (MAC) - a sedative administered through the IV to induce either conscious or unconscious sedation. It is often used for patients receiving a local or regional in order to keep them calm before and during a procedure. During conscious sedation, the patient is alert enough to respond appropriately to questions and commands. During a deeper sedation, the patient is at a less responsive level of consciousness and may no longer respond to painful or verbal stimulation.

❧❧❧

Your discussion with the anesthesiologist should take place before you have had any narcotic or hypnotic medication so that you are completely clear-headed and able to understand the explanations. It is also important to be aware that any consents you sign on the day of surgery must be signed before you receive any narcotic or anesthesia. It certainly makes sense that you want to be wide awake when signing a legal document.

To begin with, you will have an IV started. Your doctor may also have ordered an antibiotic solution to be added to your IV prior to surgery. This is not necessarily because you have an infection, but rather to prevent one. It is a prophylactic, or preventive, measure.

Next, you may receive a preoperative injection of a narcotic or a hypnotic to relax you and possibly a medication to dry up your secretions so that mucous will not drip down into your lungs while you are under the anesthesia.

At this point you will be taken to the Operating Room. There, the anesthesiologist takes over and is in charge of your overall condition while you are in surgery. He or she will administer your anesthesia. From then on, your respirations, blood pressure and heartbeat are monitored closely by the anesthesiologist.

If you have a Regional or MAC, you may be awake for part or all of the surgical procedure. In some cases, the surgeon needs you to be awake in order to see if you can respond to certain directions, or answer questions. If you are given a General anesthetic you will be asleep during your surgery and you won't remember any of it, and that is pretty much the point.

Nurse's Notes	*"Hi, David." Five-year old David's mother and father greet him in the Recovery Room.* *"Your surgery is all over," his Mom says. "Your hernia is fixed."* *"No, it's not," insists David. "I've been awake the whole time, and they didn't do anything yet!"*

❧❧❧

"Where am I? When does my surgery start?"

You look around through a haze. You are lying in a hospital bed with high side rails. You don't recognize the room or the nurse standing over you.

"You're in the Recovery Room," she smiles. *"Your surgery is all over, and you're doing fine."*

She wraps a blood pressure cuff around your arm, and inflates it. *"I'll be taking your blood pressure every 15 minutes until you're ready to go back to your room,"* she tells you.

You've been through surgery and you don't recall a thing. When you are awake (or at least arousable) and your vital signs (blood pressure, pulse, and respirations) are stable, the Recovery Room nurse will wheel you to your room. There you will be transferred to your hospital bed.

Even though you wake up each time the floor nurse speaks to you, you will still be groggy from all that medication, and will drop off to sleep easily.

The anticipation of anesthesia may make you nervous, but the waking up part is not hard. Your job is to sleep it off and let your nurses take care of you.

NOTES

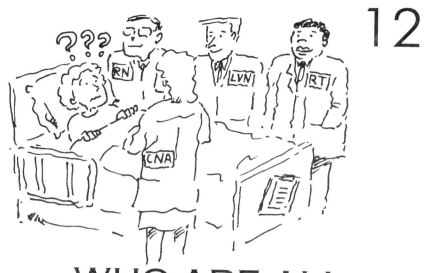

WHO ARE ALL THESE PEOPLE?

"Could you please help me to the bathroom," you ask the lady wearing dark blue pants and a light blue uniform blouse.

"I'm not the nurse," she answers. *"You must call the nurse."*

Well, you are thinking, she is wearing a uniform. So, who is she? She proceeds to bring a mop from a cart sitting in the hallway and goes to work on the floor.

With the multitude of uniform colors, solids and prints, it's hard to distinguish who's who and who does what for you and to you.

What every employee should have in common is an identification badge which states the employee's name, their license (if relevant) and department. Some hospitals include a picture on the ID badge. Some personnel are licensed, some unlicensed, but all should be wearing a badge.

If you are approached by someone who wants to do something for you or to you, it is appropriate for you to ask to see their ID badge if it is not prominently displayed on their person.

Now, who are all these people?
Let's start with the nursing staff since they will be the ones you have the most contact with. You should know from the outset that different hospitals have different dress codes, some more strict than others. Hospital A may require all nursing personnel to wear white uniforms, and a few may still insist that RN's wear caps. Hospital B may permit nurses to wear different colored uniforms, print tops, and no caps. Some allow minimal jewelry, and others permit only wedding rings. Emergency Room, Operating Room and Recovery Room personnel usually wear "scrubs," the familiar green or blue shirts and pants you see on the popular TV hospital series. Bottom line - you aren't going to be able to tell the players by their colors.

NURSING PERSONNEL

RN - Registered Nurse

The Registered Nurse has graduated from a four-year college nursing program with a Baccalaureate of Science degree (BS), or a two-year community college program with an Associate Degree (AD), or a two- or three-year hospital diploma program. Graduates from all three programs must take the same Board examinations given by their State Boards of Nursing and are entitled to call themselves Registered Nurses.

An RN will be in charge of your care at all times, a different one for each shift. These persons are responsible for planning your care from the time you are admitted to the floor until your discharge. They see that your doctor's orders are carried out, and supervise any other nursing personnel who give care to you. The RNs document your progress in your chart. They contact your doctors if any problems develop. They are responsible for coordinating treatment or services given by other departments, such as Respiratory or Physical Therapy.

If you encounter any problems during your hospitalization, the RN in charge of your care is the first person you should talk to.

LVN - Licensed Vocational Nurse or LPN - Licensed Practical Nurse

An LVN has had a one-year training course after graduation from high school. (Sometimes an entrance exam will suffice in place of a high school diploma for persons over 18). LVN courses can be taken at a community college or at a private school which trains LVN's and Nursing Assistants. Occasionally, they can be found in a high school curriculum.

These individuals, also, must pass a State Board exam.

In the hospital setting, in most states, an LVN may dispense medications, start IV's, change dressings, and may administer some treatments. In all cases, the LVN works under the direction and supervision of the RN.

Nurse's Notes	*"There you go, Mrs. Whitman." I give my patient a pat on the arm. "That pain shot should make you more comfortable real soon."* *"Thank you, Judy," she says, rolling onto her back. "Now, could you please have the Nursing Assistant come in and give me the bedpan?"* *"I can do that for you," I respond.* *"Oh no, Dear, that's not your job," she insists.* *"Taking care of you is my job," I tell her.*

In an accredited hospital, dispensing of medications and starting IV's are tasks done by licensed nurses - RNs or LVNs.

NA - Nursing Assistant or Nurse Aide, CNA - Certified Nursing Assistant

To become a Certified Nursing Assistant, an individual takes a class, anywhere from six to eighteen weeks in duration, and receives a Certificate. These classes are often given in the hospital, and are sometimes found in the local public schools.

An NA or CNA is trained to do most bedside care: giving baths, making beds, feeding patients, and assisting patients to the bathroom or with the bedpan. They take your vital signs and are trained to notice certain problems such as skin rashes or sores and changes in your condition which they then report to the RN. They can help you with many personal tasks to make you more comfortable.

Nurse's Notes	*"I didn't know orderlies were allowed to give medications," my 52-year old patient says. She is visibly upset.* *"They aren't, Mrs. Hillburn," I reply. "What happened to make you think that?"* *"On the last shift, this man instead of a nurse gave me my heart medicine," she answers. "Where are the nurses?"* *"Oh, that was Peter," I tell her. "He is an LVN."* *"I didn't know men went into nursing," she says, looking surprised.* *I make a mental note to remind Peter to identify himself to patients.*

Orderlies

Orderlies have had training in moving patients from bed to guerney, from bed to wheelchair, from guerney to OR table. These are the people who will take you to Radiology to get a chest x-ray, or to the Cardio-Vascular Lab for an angiogram.

They are not nurses, but work under the direction of your nurse when they must take you somewhere.

MEDICAL PERSONNEL

Doctors making their rounds in the hospital may or may not wear lab coats or be required to wear ID badges. If you are unclear about the identity of someone who approaches you, it's OK to say, "Tell me who you are."

Of course, you recognize your family doctor and the specialist when they make their daily rounds. But who is that young woman accompanying your doctor? She is wearing blue slacks and a white lab coat with a stethoscope sticking out of the coat pocket. Her ID badge says,

> **Laura Ramirez, M.D.**
> **Resident**

If you are in a teaching hospital, there are Residents Fellows, Interns and physicians-in-training, who may be seeing you along with your own doctors. They are well supervised by your doctors, as well as the teaching staff. You may also be assisted in your recovery by nursing students working under the supervision of an instructor.

Dr. Ramirez has completed four years of medical school, and spent a year as an intern learning the ropes on the medical and surgical floors. She rotated around to many departments, including Surgery and Pediatrics as well as the Emergency Room. Now, having decided Family Practice is where she wants to specialize, she has been accepted into a residency program and is a Family Practice Resident. She is currently working with your doctor.

OTHER LICENSED PERSONNEL

You may also encounter Physical Therapists, Dietitians, Respiratory Therapists or Social Workers. These employees are college educated and are licensed by the state. They may wear a lab coat over street clothes, or may only be wearing business attire - AND their ID badge.

ALSO APPEARING -

Housekeeping personnel will be wearing uniforms, as will engineering and other environmental workers. Any person coming into your room, whether they are there to fix your TV or unstop the toilet or to bring you a meal tray will have an ID badge, and most will be wearing a uniform.

GREY OR PINK LADIES AND GENTLEMEN

These are the dedicated men and women who give of their spare time to be hospital volunteers. They run errands for the staff, refill your water pitchers, arrange your flowers, bring you magazines and visit with you if you are lonely. Others, behind the scenes, help staff the offices, answer phones, and in countless ways keep the wheels of the hospital turning smoothly.

They usually bring smiles, too. Save one of yours for the volunteer.

ADMINISTRATION

"Hello, I'm Mary Davidson, Director of Nursing Services," the woman in a navy-blue suit smiles at you. *"I'd like to know how you're progressing and if you are satisfied with the nursing care on this floor."*

Her ID badge states her name and position. You are surprised at this visit from someone in Administration.

58

In a small hospital, this kind of personal contact might not be so rare. Administrative personnel in larger institutions, however, do not usually have time for individual visits. Their jobs are to keep the hospital up and running. Nursing is only one department, albeit the largest, which they oversee.

Budgets, fund raising, safety and legal regulations, supplies and equipment, environmental issues, and interfacing with local agencies are among the many concerns of administration.

•

Make full use of the **NOTES** pages or your note pad to keep track of the people you see each day who are involved in your hospital progress. They will be impressed that you remembered their names.

Nurse's Notes

"Here's your breakfast tray." I recognize the Nurse Aide's voice but can't see her because my eyes and much of my face are covered with bandages. I can't see the tray either. It feels strange to be on the other side of the bed. Here I am as the patient instead of the nurse. I hear the Aide's footsteps as she leaves the room.

I fumble cautiously, making my fingers creep along the closest edge of the tray. There's a bowl. It has a plastic lid. I remove the lid and put my finger in the bowl. Oh, it's very warm, gooey. I smell my finger. Oatmeal. Is there milk, sugar? Can I find something less messy?

"Can I help you?" a woman's voice, warm and gentle.

"Yes, please," I reply. "I'm afraid I'll make a mess."

This kind person takes my hand and guides me around my breakfast tray. "Here's your toast at 11 o'clock. The coffee is at 2 o'clock - it's still too hot to drink." She fixes my oatmeal and stays while I take the first bite, then she leaves. "Enjoy your breakfast." I picture her floating out of the room on angel wings.

When my nurse comes in a few minutes later, I ask her, "Who was the lady who was here just a minute ago?"

"That was our Director of Nursing," is the reply.

NOTES

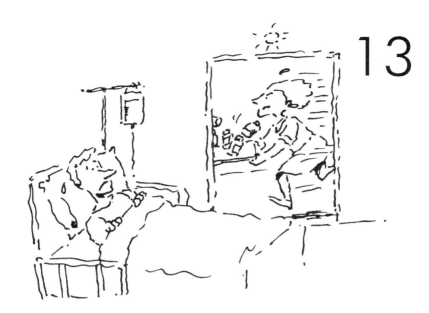

HELLO OUT THERE

"Isn't anybody ever going to take away my breakfast tray?" you wonder. The tea was weak, but nice and hot. The green jello was too green and too wiggly to deal with so early in the morning. You finally put on your call light.

"May I help you?" the secretary says over the intercom.

"Can my nurse take my tray, please?" you ask.

"The Aides are going around now picking up all the trays," she answers.

"So where is my nurse?" you grumble to yourself. *"I haven't seen her for an hour. What's she doing out there?"*

If you had X-Ray vision, here's what you would have seen since Susie Chipper, RN, came on duty at 7:00 am.

Susie listened to the report from the night nurse on you and the other six patients she will be responsible for today. She has made her first rounds and introduced herself to the patients. She gave instructions to Margaret, the

Nursing Assistant working with her today. She then checked the patients' medication records with the charts to make sure they are accurate. She has given two pain shots, and administered several IV antibiotics that were due at 8:00 am.

Morning lab results are starting to come in on the computer, and Susie has called two doctors with those results and received orders from them. One of the doctors gave orders to administer an extra dose of insulin to his patient. She writes the orders on the charts and enters the insulin order on the medication record. She then goes to the Medication Room, draws up the insulin into a syringe, and adminsters it to the patient.

On her way back to the desk, Susie sees a call light flashing outside a patient's room. She goes in to see what the patient needs.

"Oh, there you are, Susie. My dressing is coming off and there is blood on my sheets," the patient says, looking concerned. Susie reassures the patient that no harm has been done, washes her hands, puts on disposable gloves and redresses the patient's wound.

"Let me help you up to the chair," she suggests. *"You can have breakfast sitting up and we'll change your bed as soon as we can."*

Just as Susie gets back to the desk, another patient's daughter comes up to her.

"My mother got coffee on her tray, and she wanted tea," the woman complains. *"Why can't they get things right?"*

"I'm sorry. We'll get her some tea," Susie responds and then gives instructions to the Nursing Assistant to make the tea.

She completes her medication check, then begins to pass morning medications, due at 9:00. She is interrupted twice. The first time it is to assess a patient who threw up her breakfast. She gives the patient an anti-nausea medication. Then she takes a phone call from a doctor asking for a progress report on his patient.

By 10:00 o'clock, Susie has finally finished passing morning medications, and four doctors have made rounds and written new orders on their patients. She has assisted a doctor to change a dressing, and inserted a catheter into a patient who has not been able to urinate.

Each time Susie goes into a patient's room, she automatically checks whatever electronic and mechanical equipment the patient has. All six of her patients have IVs which are on controllers. One of her patients has pneumatic boots to promote good circulation in the legs. Another had knee surgery and has his leg in a mobilizer which bends his knee to a certain degree and then straightens it. Susie must regulate and monitor this equipment frequently during her shift.

"Want to go to coffee?" a co-worker asks.

"No thanks, but I can't," Susie answers. *"I have to restart an IV that isn't running right, and give two pain shots."*

"My mother hasn't had her bath yet," the daughter is back at the desk with more complaints.

"The Nursing Assistant is bathing patients now," Susie answers, *"she will be with your mother in about 15 minutes. I'll set her up to brush her teeth."* Susie sits the patient up in bed with a towel under her chin and finds her toothbrush and tooth paste in the bedside table.

"Susie," the Nursing Assistant calls from the doorway, *"Mr. Schultz is having trouble breathing."*

Susie goes to Mr. Schultz and does a quick assessment, checking his skin color and temperature. She listens to his lungs. She then puts an oxygen cannula on the patient and turns the flow to a low level.

"Stay with him," Susie instructs the Nursing Assistant, then goes to the desk to call Mr. Schultz' doctor.

And the day is just getting started. Later in the morning Susie will discharge one patient and receive another from the Intensive Care Unit. All during her shift she needs to document what is being done to and for the patients, as well as progress or lack of it. It's important for you to know that much of what she does is regulated and governed by state laws. All that paperwork is required by law or by hospital policy, and has multiplied in the last few years.

So that's what your nurse is doing out there. If you have asked for a pain shot or a cup of coffee, it is quite possible for your nurse to get so caught up with requests by doctors, or a very ill patient that she might be delayed or even forget. She's human too. Don't be hesitant about putting on your call light and asking that she be reminded.

Another tip about pain shots: don't wait until the pain is excrutiating to make your request. When you feel the pain coming on, ask your nurse for the pain medication. You will make your day go more smoothly, and hers too.

NOTES

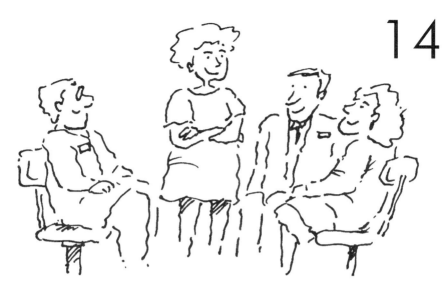

14

WHO'S IN CHARGE?

"Turn over, please. I'm going to give you a shot."

"Let me have your arm. I'm going to draw some blood."

"Your doctor ordered an X-ray. I'm taking you to Radiology."

Wait a minute. What's in the shot? Why is my blood being drawn? My doctor didn't tell me anything about an X-ray.

You, the well-informed reader, are not going to be intimidated by a uniform and an authoritative voice. Though you realize that the nurses and technicians are carrying out your doctor's orders, you also know that you have a right to be informed about any procedure that is to be done to you. It's your body, and you are in charge of it.

"Before I turn over, tell me what's in the syringe and what it's for." "Is that what the doctor ordered for me?"

"What blood tests did my doctor order? My name is Mary Wells. Do you have the right patient?"

"My doctor didn't mention an X-ray. Will you please double-check with my nurse."

If your doctor has ordered daily medications for you, your nurse will bring them at the times prescribed. Usually, they will be handed to you in a little white paper cup along with a cup of water. It's OK for you to ask the nurse to explain what you are being given and what each one is for.

"The blood pressure pill I take at home is pink. This one is blue. Are you sure it's the right one?"

That is a reasonable question. The answer may be that your doctor is prescribing a different dosage during your illness, or that the hospital uses a different brand than the one dispensed by your pharmacist. It's OK to pose these questions. It's important that you do. Mistakes can and do happen. Even the most skilled doctor or nurse can make errors. It's rare, but it happens. You can be the double-checker, to make sure everything done to you is meant for you, and that any questions you have are answered.

What about those days and nights when you are groggy from medication or feeling lousy with nausea and pain? That's when you may need an advocate — a friend or family member who can stay with you.

With the advent of managed care, doctors have more patients to see each day. When your doctors make rounds, you and your advocate can help them make the most efficient use of their time with you by making sure that they are informed of your needs and address all your concerns.

During this period of recovery, it will be a big help if your advocate can be in the room to ask the nurses and technicians to explain what they are doing. It's also useful to have an extra hand to give you a sip of water, close the blinds, or help you with your meals. Of course, this person would not do any nursing care or intrude on the nurses' activities. He or she would be there as friend (or intermediary), not a replacement to the nursing staff.

The best way to insure that you get what you need, and have the best possible hospital stay, is to encourage an advocate to be present and speak up for you. Ask, before admission to the hospital, about the policies on someone staying with you.

Following Orders

You have asked your doctors and your surgeon to find out what's wrong with you and to fix it. They will use their best professional judgment in deciding the course of treatment. It is important to be able to trust your physicians to keep you informed and answer your questions honestly.

So here you are, in the hospital, flat on your back. You've picked your surgeon, had your surgery, and are in the process of recovering. Who's in charge?

It's a shared responsibility. Your physicians are in charge of your overall medical care. The nurses are responsible for carrying out the doctor's orders, observing your response to the various treatments, reporting any problems to the doctor, and documenting your progress. So what's left for you to do?

You can help the doctors and nurses by sharing your observations, and by staying informed about your plan of care. It really amounts to being aware of how your body is reacting to whatever is going on and reporting these reactions to the nurse and the doctor.

"Hello, Mrs. Lockhart," John, the nurse, addresses your roommate. *"How are you feeling today?"* he asks. You listen for the elderly woman's answer.

"So, how should I feel? I had surgery - see they cut me here in the belly," she whimpers.

"How do you think I feel? What are you? Some kind of newspaper reporter? I feel lousy!"

You try not to laugh out loud. (It would hurt too much to laugh!) The nurse finishes his examination of Mrs. Lockhart. It's your turn. You're a smart cookie. You've read this book cover to cover and you're ready for him.

"Hi there," he says, turning to you. *"How are you doing today?"*

"Hello, John. Well, I had a lot of pain around my incision today, and the evening nurse gave me a shot. It helped a lot. But now it's starting to hurt again. And, by the way, the nausea is back—but only when I try to turn over."

You have just given this nurse more information than you realize. He knows how long it has been since your last pain shot, so he can assess if the dosage is adequate. He suspects that the nausea you are experiencing is not from the narcotic in the pain shot, but probably a residual effect of anesthesia. You have also given him the important information that you are able to move adequately to at least make the attempt to change your position.

John explains to you about the anesthetic, and says that he will bring you an injection with a combination of pain and nausea reliever.

"I am glad to see you moving yourself in the bed," he adds. *"It is very important for you to move all your extremities (arms and legs). It keeps your circulation going."*

Now, he comes in with a shocking piece of news.

"After your pain shot has taken effect, I am going to help you sit on the edge of the bed and we'll take a little walk. That will help to strengthen your muscles. It won't be easy," he continues, *"but I'll be right here to assist you."*

You are tempted to repeat Mrs. Lockhart's plaintive cry, *"You don't understand - I just had surgery. Right here, in my belly."* But you don't.

Later that night you have several questions bouncing around in your head. Maybe you are wondering when you can eat solid food, or when you can go back to work. Clever reader, you have read *Take It Or Leave It* and have your note pad and pencil handy. So you make yourself a note of questions to ask your doctor when he makes rounds.

Your physician makes rounds once a day while you're in the hospital, more if you are in critical condition. After he has left your bedside and probably the hospital, you don't want to be left with burning issues like, *"What if I can't have a normal bowel movement?"* and *"Can I take a shower today?"* When he or she walks into your hospital room and says, *"How are you doing today?"* don't feel self-conscious about picking up your note pad and saying, *"I'm glad it's over, and it hurts like heck, and I have a few questions."* This is the time to say, *"The pain medication doesn't hold me very long. Can you do something about that?"* or *"I'm so thirsty. When can I have something to drink?"*

Include on your list of questions for the doctor inquiries about lab test results, how the surgery went, what he found and how soon you can get out of this place (not that you feel like sprinting down the hall right this minute). Remember, your questions are reasonable. You have a right to reasonable answers. It's your body. Only you can feel the inside.

So **who's in charge?**

It's a shared responsibility. When doctors and nurses ask you questions, give them specific answers. This helps everyone do his/her job which is taking care of you.

The most important aspect of your job is taking part in your own recovery. Listen to the instructions the nurses and therapists give you pertaining to your exercises, how to take your medications, activities to avoid. Be good to yourself when you go home. Follow the doctor's orders about rest and diet. Take care of this vehicle which is your body. What you do to it, what you put into it, what you allow to be done to it has an effect. This really is the first day of the rest of your life. And *you're in charge.*

NOTES

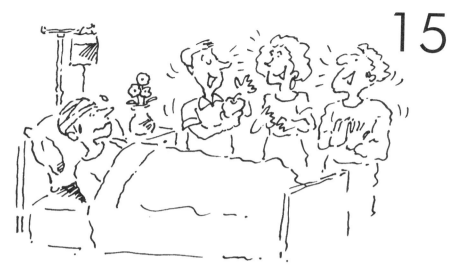

VISITORS - GUIDELINES

Ah, yes. You've just been helped into bed by the nurse after a walk in the hall. You sink back into your pillow with a grateful sigh. Now, for a little nap.

"Hi, there!" You are startled awake by a hearty voice. *"We thought we'd all come and cheer you up!"*

It's the gang from the office. Six smiling co-workers ring your bed, some holding huge bouquets of flowers, others handing you boxes tied with ribbons.

"It's See's candies - your favorite, chocolate covered marshmallows."

"Where can I put these flowers? Are there any vases here?"

They're such good friends. You don't want to hurt their feelings, BUT...

How can you let your friends know if and when you would like to have visitors? A little advance communication

71

is a good start. If you hate having people around you when you are sick, let everyone know ahead of time that you'll be open to visitors after you're home and feeling better. If you would be comforted by seeing caring friends you could let them know that.

"Perhaps you could come by for a short visit. I find that I tire very quickly, but I would love to see you."

Here are some useful Guidelines for your prospective visitors. Add some of your own ideas, thoughts on the **NOTES** page at the end of this chapter. Before you are admitted to the hospital you might want to leave this book in a prominent place at work, open to this page!

❦❦❦

VISITORS, PLEASE:

- Check with a family member or close friend to see if the patient would like to have visitors. If he is the type who would honestly rather suffer in solitude, do respect his wishes.
- Call the hospital to inquire about visiting hours. If the hours are noon to 8:00 p.m., don't pop in unexpectedly for a surprise visit at 10:00 a.m. You might surprise the patient in the middle of a bath. If the patient is in an intensive care unit, visitors might not be permitted except for family members or a significant other. Visiting hours for family might be more flexible in these units. Call the hospital first.
- If you want to bring flowers, make sure the patient is not allergic to them. Keep the bouquet small. Patient rooms are limited in counter or table top space. Choose a potted plant, or if you bring cut flowers, include a vase. Another possibility is to send or bring flowers to the home after your friend is discharged.

- Short visits are best - ten to twenty minutes. That's ample time to let him know that you care and find out if he needs anything. However, if your friend indicates that he really wants you to stay and talk or just keep him company, by all means pull up a chair.
- Visit in small groups - two or three people at the most.
- Rather than calling the Nurses' Station to find out how your friend is doing, call the family to get an update. Nurses are permitted to give out only general information to non-family.
- If your friend has a roommate, be respectful of his privacy. He might be resting or trying to watch TV. Speak quietly. Ask the roommate if he would like the curtain between the two beds closed.
- Perhaps you are someone who is really uncomfortable around hospitals and sick people. Or maybe you don't know the patient well enough to pay a visit. That's OK. You don't have to show up in person to let your friend know that you are concerned. Patients like getting cards and notes.
- It's better not to bring food as a gift unless you know that the patient is allowed to have it. The doctor may have ordered that your friend is NPO (nothing by mouth), or is limited as to salt, sugar or fibrous foods.
- Don't plan to bring your friend his favorite martini. It might not mix too well with his medications. Gift wrap a jar of olives for later use at home instead.
- If you have a cold, cough or flu, stay home, drink lots of fluids and keep your bugs to yourself. Your friend has enough problems without you.
- Try not to bring infants or very small children with you. Considering the multitude of bacteria and viruses, hospitals are not great places for susceptible little ones.

There are a few exceptions. One might be an Obstetrics unit where siblings are allowed to visit a new baby brother or sister. In another case, family might arrange to bring a nursing infant in to a mother hospitalized with an unrelated medical problem. A third exception would be a child who is distraught over Daddy or Grandma being in the hospital, and who would be reassured if only he might see for himself that everything is OK and get a big hug. In this case, the family could ask the nurse if there is a lounge where the patient could be brought to have a visit with the child.

- It can be uncomfortable, even painful, for the patient if visitors sit or lean on his bed.
- If this is a 2-bed room and the other bed is vacant, don't sit on or lay your coats and purses on the empty bed. It must be kept clean for the next patient. Ask the nurse for an extra chair.

Nurse's Notes	*I enter the patient's room carrying a tray of sterile dressing supplies. I am shocked to see a visitor changing her baby's diaper on the empty bed.* *"Oh nurse," the lady says with a bright smile, "can you please get me a wash cloth?"*

- If you need to use the bathroom, ask someone where the public restrooms are. Patient bathrooms are for their use only .
- Don't talk about your aches and pains or your Uncle Joe who had the same surgery and ended up paralyzed.
- You might be visiting during your lunch break, but eat your pastrami sandwich before you come in to the hospital. Strong food odors make some people nauseated when they are not feeling well.

- Your friend may or may not feel like talking about his surgery or illness. Let him guide the conversation. And, by all means, don't suggest treatments that he could have sought if only he had asked you, the medical guru.

Thank you, Visitors, for following these guidelines. Your friend will appreciate your thoughtfulness.

If you are looking for something to bring the patient other than flowers or candy, here are some suggestions:

Gift Ideas for the Hospitalized Patient

- A magazine your friend doesn't usually see.
- The loan of your Walkman and several music tapes or Books on Tape, or a portable CD player with discs.
- A pretty box of note cards with the envelopes already stamped (include a pen).
- A current TV guide.
- A pair of outrageous socks for keeping feet warm at night. Go crazy - get something with a wild design.
- Have everyone at the office sign a "Get Well Soon" card.
- A box of body powder or hand lotion.
- Anything hand-made by a child.
- A gift certificate good for a personally-delivered home-cooked meal when the patient goes home.
- The daily paper.

🌹🌹🌹

Your friends and family mean well, and these guidelines will help them to do well. Later, when a friend of yours is hospitalized, you will be a model visitor. When that happens, be sure to give her a copy of this book.

NOTES

16

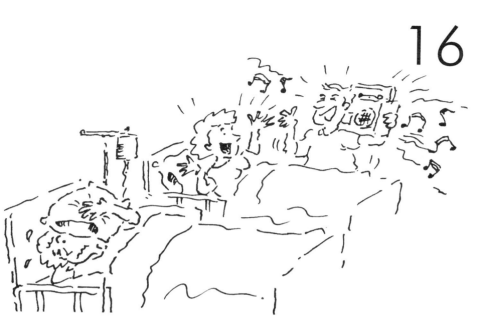

DOUBLE
OCCUPANCY

"What is that awful noise?" A sound like a buzzsaw jolts you awake. Oh no! It's your roommate snoring! You realize with dismay that you are not going to get much sleep. This is one of the downsides of a semi-private room. For the next few days you will be sharing not only your "bedroom" but your bathroom with a perfect stranger. Not a normal situation!

It really is asking a lot to expect two people who never laid eyes on each other before to share such intimate facilities. When you add the fact that they are both ill, having tests, bathroom accidents, etc. — it's amazing that it can work at all.

Surviving a roommate is possible and requires a special *Take It and Leave It* list.

TAKE IT

1. Ear plugs and eye mask to give yourself a little audio and visual privacy. Ear plugs can keep snoring and general hospital noises somewhat muffled. An eye mask in addition to shutting out light gives a clear signal that you don't feel like chatting.
2. A portable radio with earphones to provide your choice of entertainment and to tune out unwanted noise or conversation.
3. A little extra tolerance and plenty of tact. The Golden Rule and common courtesy go a long way in getting along with a roommate.

LEAVE IT

1. False pride. No one looks his best while a patient in the hospital. So your hair is a mess. Don't worry about it. You're a patient, you're sick, you're entitled.
2. Timidity. If there is a problem with your roommate it really is OK to speak to the person directly or to the nurse.

Visitors can be a problem at times. If your roommate has too many at one time or if they stay too long, speak to the nurse. If you need to go to the bathroom and will need to struggle past the visitors in your designer gown, ask them to step outside for a few minutes or ask the nurse to make the request.

You will have the most privacy if you have a window bed, though in some hospitals that puts you farther from the bathroom. If you don't get your preference at first ask the nurse to move you at the earliest opportunity.

When you get a new roommate introduce yourself. It's good to be friendly and at the same time you want to keep a certain personal space between you. You don't need to give all the details of your medical situation. "I had abdominal surgery and hope to go home in two days" is a sufficient explanation.

You can be very helpful in orienting your new roommate to the hospital routine, and especially to the TV. This is a great opportunity to explain the volume control knob, and to point out that later at night the speaker can be kept close to the ear with the volume turned down. If your roommate misses the point and tends to have the TV on too loud and too late, ask the nurse to handle the problem.

You might get a roommate who is confused and constantly tries to get out of bed, causing you to keep calling for the nurse. Another possibility is someone who yells out all night long. These people usually can't help their behavior, but that is no reason for you to feel you have to watch out for them. You also should not have to be kept awake all night by the yelling or by your concern for the other patient. You are in the hospital to get well. Ask to speak to the Charge Nurse. Tell her your concerns for the safety of your roommate and at the same time ask for a room change. Helpful hint: It's best to make your request for a room change early in the day.

Privacy and confidentiality are difficult to maintain in a semi-private room. If you overhear intimate or confidential conversations going on at your roommate's bedside (e.g. a doctor discussing test results) put on your earphones and listen to some music. If your doctor or nurse begins to discuss something about you that you don't want overheard and if you are able to be up, ask if there is somewhere more private where you could talk. You have a right to privacy regarding your medical situation.

These suggestions may help you to be a first-rate, certainly a forewarned, roommate. You may even discover that you enjoy having a fellow patient to talk to.

NOTES

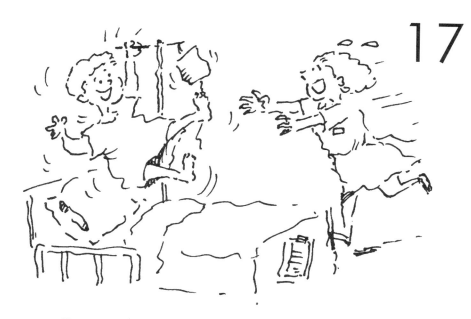

CHILDREN, BABIES, AND HOSPITALS

"I went to the hospital and had surgery," five-year old David proudly points to his bandage. *"And I got new Legos,"* he continues.

"My Mommy is getting me a baby sister," four-year old Charles proclaims, *"and I get to hold her."*

"Daddy went to the hospital, and maybe he won't come back," three-year old Jonathan says, tears running down his cheeks.

"I have a breastfeeding infant at home," the young mother tells her nurse, *"and here I am — stuck in the hospital with a broken leg."*

All of these scenarios call for education before and during hospitalization.

81

David came through his hernia operation with flying colors, because his parents did their homework. How parents prepare themselves and the child for surgery will be tailor-made for the situation and the child. Parents are urged to go to the library or bookstore and look up the many fine books for adults and children on these subjects. Mr. Rogers' book is one of the best. (See the References and Resources for other suggestions.) If possible, take the child to visit the hospital beforehand. Preparation pays off.

Telling the child what to expect on a level he can understand can be helpful in reducing fear. It is also important to give the child time to ask questions and to provide honest answers.

> *"Is the shot going to hurt?"*
> *"Yes, but only for a moment and then it will stop."*

Your child may need to talk or draw or play about some of the feelings he is experiencing.

What if your child has to stay one or more nights in the hospital? Is it OK to ask your pediatrician or the surgeon if you can arrange to stay overnight in the room? You bet! If Hospital A doesn't make such provisions, ask your doctor what other options you have.

Little Charles would enjoy a special class for big brothers and sisters. Find out if your hospital has one.

He will learn how to hold the new baby, the importance of washing his hands, and how to play with the baby.

In the case of three-year old Jonathan, he might not be consoled until he can see for himself that Daddy is all right. Ask the doctor and the floor nurses if there is a way for Jonathan to visit his father. Explain to the child in advance what he will see.

> *"Daddy is lying in his own special bed. He has little tubes placed in his nose (oxygen) to help him breathe better. He's been sick and is kind of tired, but he can't wait to see you. Let's make him a get well card."*

If it is not possible for the child to come to the hospital, get him involved in planning for Daddy's homecoming. Make a big Welcome sign, bake cookies, put extra pillows on the sofa to make Daddy comfy. This will give Jonathan tangible evidence that his father is coming back.

The breastfeeding mother has a unique situation that calls for special measures. It is possible for the mother to keep up her milk supply by pumping. If the mother does plan to use a pump while in the hospital, a family member or close friend should plan to stay in the room to assist her. In some cases the milk can be fed to the infant by the caregiver at home (depending on the medications the mother is taking). This would need to be discussed in advance with the Pediatrician. Ask if the hospital has a Lactation Specialist who can consult with the mother and her doctor.

Another excellent resource for the breastfeeding mother is La Leche League. As soon as it is known that hospitalization is required, the mother can contact LLL 1-800-LA LECHE for referral to a local group Leader. An accredited LLL Leader can provide information to help you understand what some of your choices are while you are hospitalized.

There is help out there for mothers who are separated from their babies, but wish to continue breastfeeding. It takes a little extra effort, but it is definitely worth it. See the References and Resources listed at the back of the book for some expert advice.

Babies and children aren't necessarily incompatible with hospitals. It just takes some research on your part to understand your options, and a determination to make it work.

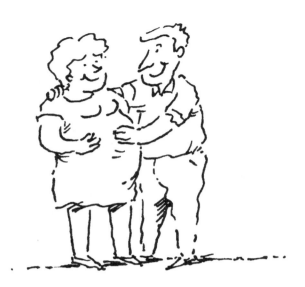

Childbirth

You're expecting and you're looking forward to motherhood, but you're not sure what to expect in the hospital. Well, you're in luck! Most of the sections of this book pertain to you just as easily as to someone who is being hospitalized for hip surgery. The major difference is in the length of your hospital stay. You may go home the same day or you may stay one or two days.

Several months before your due date, you may want to discuss with your obstetrician the type of anesthesia that will be used, if any. At that time you could discuss the option to have significant family members present at the birth. Doing some reading on childbirth and becoming educated about various options can go a long way toward having the kind of birth you want. You may want to write a Birth Plan and go over this with your doctor. When the questions of tests, ultrasound, or hospital procedures come up, you can discuss the pros and cons for you, so that you have a clear understanding of the risks and benefits, before agreeing with his suggestions.

Some hospitals offer free tours and classes for prospective parents. Take advantage of them. The Head Nurse on the Labor and Delivery floor would be a good person to talk to. You may want to see if you can make an appointment with her, and bring along your notes or Birth Plan. Discuss your preferences with her. Is rooming-in an option? If so, she may want to know which family member will stay in the room while you sleep. Or is it all right for the baby to stay in the nursery at times?

If you plan to breastfeed your baby, and you don't want the baby to be given any supplements or artificial nipples, you need to make this clear in your discussion with her and in your Birth Plan. All these things can and should be talked out in advance.

If you are uncomfortable with some of the hospital's policies, you are free to ask if they are flexible. See where you can compromise. If you are still not comfortable about this hospital's policies, ask your obstetrician if you have another choice of hospitals.

If you plan to breastfeed, La Leche League offers classes and support. Attending a few of their meetings before your baby's birth can provide you with much information and maybe even new friends.

See the References and Resources section for some excellent books to help you plan for the birth of your baby. It's a very important event in your life, and worth a little research.

If you don't know your options, you don't have any!

NOTES

18

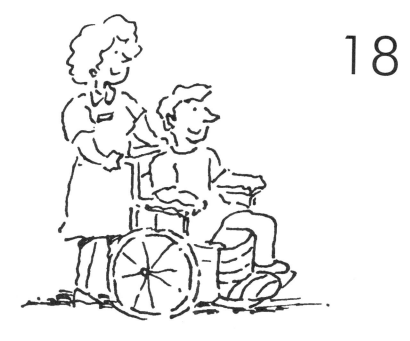

HOW DO I GET OUT OF THIS PLACE?

"Oh no!" you moan. *"Not more paperwork!"* Your nurse has just come in with several sheets of paper. *"My doctor said I could go home,"* you point out.

"You are discharged," she assures you. *"I just have a few things to go over with you."*

Your nurse is being thorough. She will go over your doctor's instructions for at-home care, including activity and diet restrictions. She will make sure you understand how and when to take your medications.

Nurse's Notes	*I have looked everywhere and still can't find my patient. Dr. Post discharged him and left instructions and prescriptions on the chart. Now, where is that guy? Not in the bathroom; not in the visitors' lounge. I decide to call his house. He answers the phone.* *"Mr. Fellows," I say, trying to stay calm, "This is your nurse. I've been looking all over for you."* *"Well," he says, "the doctor said I could go home - so I did!"*

Once your physician has said that he is releasing you, your nurse holds the key to your escape. Do give her a chance to complete the paperwork. Some of the information might even be useful.

When your doctor tells you that you can go home, ask if your prescriptions will be filled at the hospital or if you must have them filled at an outside pharmacy. If it is the latter perhaps he can phone them in so that you can pick them up on the way home. (Have your pharmacist's phone number handy.) Another possibility is to have him give you the prescriptions the day before discharge so that a family member or friend can have them filled for you.

Now your job is to go on a search and rescue mission. Search every drawer for your belongings. Greeting cards and combs have a way of falling into small nooks. Can't find your slippers? Try under the bed - a favorite hiding place. Ask the Nursing Assistant to help you.

When your nurse gives you the GO sign, and your friend has arrived to take you home, you are ready for the royal chariot. The Nursing Assistant or a Volunteer will wheel you out in style in a wheelchair. (Exceptions can be made for patients who have had hemorrhoid surgery!)

"Goodbye," you say to Nurse Chipper, *"Thanks for everything."* Your smile is rueful as you recall the shots in the rear, her unrelenting insistence that you walk in the hall in spite of excruciating pain, and being served green jello three days in a row. Then you remember the gentle hands repositioning you in bed and straightening your blankets. You remember the reassuring voice when you weren't sure you could make it to the bathroom. *"Thank you, Nurse Chipper,"* you wave, and your smile is genuine.

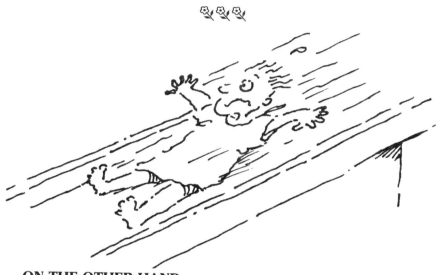

ON THE OTHER HAND...

"What do you mean I'm going home tomorrow?" you say to your doctor. *"I'm still having pain in my incision!"*

What if you feel that you are being discharged too soon? This is a subject that must be discussed with your doctor in advance of your discharge. Are you being discharged because your doctor feels that you are ready to go home, or because your health plan or the hospital utilization committee has set a limit on the number of days you may stay? Physicians have a duty to do what's best for you, but sometimes they are pressured by hospital or insurance company restrictions.

You can be prepared to speak up for yourself if you feel your discharge is premature.

There are some good reasons for patients being sent home earlier these days. Lying in bed all day is not always in your best interests. That's how some patients develop pneumonia. At home you will be more active which is actually good for you. Besides, a hospital is not a place to get a good night's sleep. If the nurses are not waking you to take your blood pressure or change your IV, they are ministering to your roommate.

The physician's point of view is, in general, that patients shouldn't be discharged if they're still suffering from fever, confusion or disorientation, inability to take liquids by mouth, faintness or inability to get to the bathroom without help. If you were hospitalized with an infection and are still running a fever, you are right to question the discharge. If you were admitted with chest pain (angina) and a heart attack was ruled out, has the reason for the chest pain been explained to you?

If you feel that your discharge is premature discuss it with your doctor and the hospital's discharge planner. If you still feel that you are being sent home too soon, ask what the appeal process is. Write a note to the director of the hospital or your health plan's director, stating specifically why you feel you should not be discharged at this time. Have a family member deliver the note personally.

Your reluctance to go home may be due to concerns about how you are going to get along at home - difficulty bathing or fixing meals, for example. Perhaps you will need to change your surgical dressing and are nervous about that. Ask the discharge planner or hospital social worker about the possibility of having a licensed nurse come to the house to change the dressing. Ask about having a home health aide come to assist with bathing. Find out about Meals on Wheels. The key to an appropriate discharge is communication with your doctor, the discharge planner and your family.

NOTES

NOTES

19

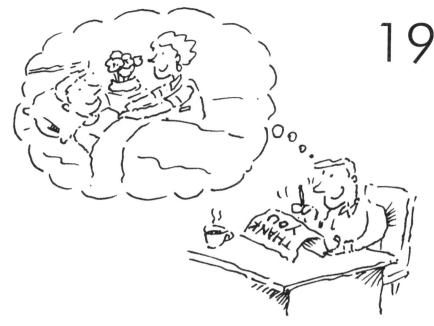

HOW CAN I EVER THANK YOU? OR SHOULD I?

"You've all been wonderful. Thank you so much. Goodbye. Thank you."

You wave as you are wheeled down the hall toward the elevator. Saying 'thank you' somehow doesn't seem adequate when you recall the care and attention you have received during your five days in the hospital. Your doctors have been so attentive. Some of the nurses found time to stay and talk with you when you were having a bad night. The orderly was so gentle as he helped move you from your bed to the OR guerney. You hope you remembered to thank all of them.

Well, you did, and they appreciated it. A simple 'thank you' means a lot.

What if you want to do more? There are several ways to show your appreciation to nurses and hospital staff.

<table>
<tr><td>

Nurse's Notes

</td><td>

"Ooh, chocolates! Who gave these to us?"
"Mrs. Wells who had the colon surgery left these for all the staff."
"How nice! Save me a caramel!"

</td></tr>
</table>

Candy is dandy and a letter is better. Nurses love candy, but a letter to the Nursing Administrator lasts longer. If you want to single out a particular nurse or other employee and let the Administrator or Head Nurse know of your appreciation, a personal note mentioning the employee by name will be passed on to the individual in addition to going into the person's file. Be assured, these letters are prized. Make it short and state what it was that impressed you or how that person made your stay less stressful.

"The night nurse, Doris, sat and talked with me when I couldn't get comfortable. I know she was busy, but she made time for me."

"Marina was my nurse for several days, and she really helped me understand the nature of my illness."

"Janie, the nursing assistant, was so patient. She fed me my soup when I just didn't have the energy."

Doctors appreciate letters too. Drop a short note to your doctors just to say thanks for getting you through all this.

Another way of saying "thank you" is to do it in advance.

Nurse's Notes	*The orderly wheels my daughter swiftly down the hall and into the Labor and Delivery section. She is doubled over with a contraction.* *Once the nurse has her settled into a bed my daughter takes a package out of her tote bag and gives it to the nurse.* *"Well," she says, "I wanted to thank you in advance, so I made you some brownies."*

No matter how you choose to say thank you, it will be appreciated.

🌹🌹🌹

Where is the Complaint Department?

Hospital administrators really do want to know about problems you encounter during your stay. If possible, make your concerns known while you are still there. Start by talking to the nurse in charge of your care or your physician, depending on the problem.

If it has to do with nursing care, employee performance, or hospital policies, talk to your nurse. If she is not able to help you resolve it, ask to speak to the Head Nurse or a Supervisor. Use a positive approach.

"I wouldn't want you to do anything that goes against your policies, Nurse Chipper. So, who else could I speak to about this? Perhaps the Head Nurse can help me."

If your concern has to do with the medical management of your care, orders which your physician has written, or plans for your date of discharge, bring it up to your primary care doctor or surgeon.

Most hospitals have a Patient Ombudsman or Patient Relations Director. These people are there specifically to help you with problems related to your hospitalization. Discussing your upset or concern at the time can keep small problems from becoming big ones. Sometimes it is just a matter of your explaining to a nurse what your preferences are. Other times, you might be less concerned if you have things explained to you.

If problems don't get resolved, or if you still feel after your discharge that they should be brought to someone's attention, write a letter to Nursing Administration or Hospital Administration.

Perhaps they will even thank you.

NOTES

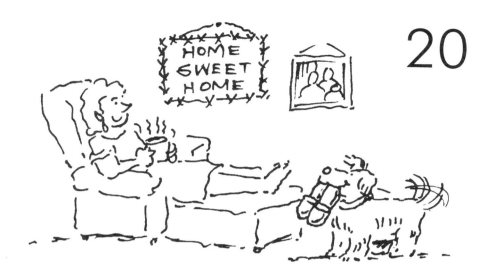

20

HOME, SWEET HOME

"It feels so good to be home," you sigh as you sink (slowly) into your favorite chair. *"I hope I don't have to do this again very soon!"*

Now, you can get on with your life. And who's in charge? **That's right - You Are.**

You've had quite an education during the last few days. You are now an experienced and more knowledgeable hospital patient. Use that knowledge to keep you on a track of well-being.

For the immediate future follow the physician's instructions. You have asked him what complications might arise, and you will call him if you have any concerns. Of course, you'll follow the medication directions and keep your office appointments.

You probably will tire more easily than you had anticipated. Don't try to get back into your usual activities right away. You might have spurts of energy, but don't be fooled. Start out with baby steps, increasing the time and energy gradually. Take frequent breaks.

Now is a good time to review your lifestyle. Since you have had a significant break in your daily routine this is an ideal time to make a fresh start. Here are five lifestyle changes for you to consider:

1. Clean out your refrigerator. Has your diet been partially responsible for your medical problems? How about going for lower fat intake? Smaller portions? More fruits and vegies? Talk it over with your primary care doctor.
2. How about exercise? Get a few friends or neighbors to join you in a "walking club." (Remember - start out slowly.)
3. Want to stop smoking? You have a head start since you probably weren't allowed to smoke in the hospital room. Each time you start to reach for a cigarette do something with your hands instead. Reorganize your desk drawer, clean out a cupboard or write a letter. Look for a smoking cessation class.
4. Take time out each day to give your busy brain a rest. Relax with some good music or spend time digging in the garden.
5. Relaxation techniques are wonderful tools for dealing with anxiety and tension. Use the exercises you practiced before going into the hospital. A favorite is TADB. Take A Deep Breath. Take two, they're easy. Close your eyes and inhale, nice and slow. Then exhale slowly and completely. Repeat as needed.

Dean Ornish's book (see References and Resources) is a wonderful source for relaxation and meditation techniques, diet changes (including recipes) and new directions in lifestyle.

Do you have a new diagnosis of a chronic disease, e.g. Lupus or Diabetes? Or perhaps a new colostomy to learn to deal with? There are support groups for just about every kind of medical problem where you can learn first-hand how other people cope. You can also be a support to others. Ask your doctor about these groups, or inquire at your hospital's Social Services department.

Many physicians and nurses feel that patients who are informed and have positive attitudes and trust their doctors seem to heal more quickly than those who arrive at the hospital full of tension and doubts. Some studies have shown that positive emotions boost the immune system. Asking questions and keeping yourself informed will go a long way toward reassuring you and keeping you in a positive frame of mind.

Do you have a Mr. Gloom among your friends? Someone who always sees and fears the worst in any situation? Try to keep your contact with Mr. G. to a minimum. When he brings up examples of people he knows who had terrible complications with your type of surgery or medical problem, change the subject and tell him some jokes. Maybe you can make him laugh. Laughter is good therapy for both of you.

These tips are just a start. You know better than anyone how you can improve the quality of your life.

You've come a long way. You've learned more than you ever wanted to know about hospitals. Hopefully, they are not as intimidating to you now. You've been there. Congratulations! You didn't just survive. You became a full partner in your own health care.

NOTES

A Patient's Bill of Rights

A Patient's Bill of Rights was first adopted by the American Hospital Association in 1973. This revision was approved by the AHA Board of Trustees on October 21, 1992.

The American Hospital Association presents *A Patient 's Bill of Rights* with the expectation that it will contribute to more effective patient care and be supported by the hospital on behalf of the institution, its medical staff, employees, and patients. The American Hospital Association encourages health care institutions to tailor this bill of rights to their patient community by translating and/or simplifying the language of this bill of rights as may be necessary to ensure that patients and their families understand their rights and responsibilities.

Bill of Rights[1]

1. The patient has the right to considerate and respectful care.

2. The patient has the right to and is encouraged to obtain from physicians and other direct caregivers relevant, current, and understandable information concerning diagnosis, treatment, and prognosis.

Except in emergencies when the patient lacks decision-making capacity and the need for treatment is urgent, the patient is entitled to the opportunity to discuss and request information related to the specific procedures and/or treatments, the risks involved, the possible length of recuperation, and the medically reasonable alternatives and their accompanying risks and benefits.

---

[1] These rights can be exercised on the patient's behalf by a designated surrogate or proxy decision maker if the patient lacks decision-making capacity, is legally incompetent, or is a minor.

Patients have the right to know the identity of physicians, nurses, and others involved in their care, as well as when those involved are students, residents, or other trainees. The patient also has the right to know the immediate and long-term financial implications of treatment choices, insofar as they are known.

3. The patient has the right to make decisions about the plan of care prior to and during the course of treatment and to refuse a recommended treatment or plan of care to the extent permitted by law and hospital policy and to be informed of the medical consequences of this action.

In case of such refusal, the patient is entitled to other appropriate care and services that the hospital provides or transfer to another hospital. The hospital should notify patients of any policy that might affect patient choice with the institution.

4. The patient has the right to have an advance directive (such as a living will, health care proxy, or durable power of attorney for health care) concerning treatment or designating a surrogate decision maker with the expectation that the hospital will honor the intent of that directive to the extent permitted by law and hospital policy.

Health care institutions must advise patients of their rights under state law and hospital policy to make informed medical choices, ask if the patient has an advance directive, and include that information in patient records. The patient has the right to timely information about hospital policy that may limit its ability to implement fully a legally valid advance directive.

5. The patient has the right to every consideration of privacy. Case discussion, consultation, examination, and treatment should be conducted so as to protect each patient's privacy.

6. The patient has the right to expect that all communications and records pertaining to his/her care will be treated as confidential by the hospital, except in cases such as suspected abuse and public health hazards when reporting is permitted or required by law. The patient has the right to expect that the hospital will emphasize the confidentiality of this information when it releases it to any other parties entitled to review information in these records.

7. The patient has the right to review the records pertaining to his/her medical care and to have the information explained or interpreted as necessary, except when restricted by law.

8. The patient has the right to expect that, within its capacity and policies, a hospital will make reasonable response to the request of a patient for appropriate and medically indicated care and services. The hospital must provide evaluation, service, and/or referral as indicated by the urgency of the case. When medically appropriate and legally permissible, or when a patient has so requested, a patient may be transferred to another facility. The institution to which the patient is to be transferred must first have accepted the patient for transfer. The patient must also have the benefit of complete information and explanation concerning the need for, risks, benefits, and alternatives to such a transfer.

9. The patient has the right to ask and be informed of the existence of business relationships among the

hospital, educational institutions, other health care providers, or payers that may influence the patient's treatment and care.

10. The patient has the right to consent to or decline to participate in proposed research studies or human experimentation affecting care and treatment or requiring direct patient involvement, and to have those studies fully explained prior to consent. A patient who declines to participate in research or experimentation is entitled to the most effective care that the hospital can otherwise provide.

11. The patient has the right to expect reasonable continuity of care when appropriate and to be informed by physicians and other caregivers of available and realistic patient care options when hospital care is no longer appropriate.

12. The patient has the right to be informed of hospital policies and practices that relate to patient care, treatment, and responsibilities. The patient has the right to be informed of available resources for resolving disputes, grievances, and conflicts, such as ethics committees, patient representatives, or other mechanisms available in the institution. The patient has the right to be informed of the hospital's charges for services and available payment methods.

The collaborative nature of health care requires that patients, or their families/surrogates, participate in their care. The effectiveness of care and patient satisfaction with the course of treatment depend, in part, on the patient fulfilling certain responsibilities. Patients are responsible for providing information about past illnesses, hospitalizations, medications, and other matters related to health status. To participate effectively in decision making, patients must be encouraged to take responsibility for requesting additional information or clarification about their health status or treatment when they do not fully understand information and instructions. Patients are also responsible for ensuring that the health care institution has a copy of their written advance directive if they have one. Patients are responsible for informing their physicians and other caregivers if they anticipate problems in following prescribed treatment.

Patients should also be aware of the hospital's obligation to be reasonably efficient and equitable in providing care to other patients and the community. The hospital's rules and regulations are designed to help the hospital meet this obligation. Patients and their families are responsible for meeting reasonable accommodations to the needs of the hospital, other patients, medical staff, and hospital employees. Patients are responsible for providing necessary information for insurance claims and for working with the hospital to make payment arrangements, when necessary.

A person's health depends on much more than health care services. Patients are responsible for recognizing the impact of their life-style on their personal health.

A PATIENT'S BILL OF RIGHTS reprinted with permission of the American Hospital Association, copyright 1992.

NOTES

REFERENCES AND RESOURCES

Advance Directive

Shape Your Health Care Future With Health Care Advance Directives, (D15803), written with the American Bar Association and the American Medical Association, combines the living will and health-care power-of-attorney into a single form designed to meet the requirements of most state laws. Send $2 check or money order for shipping and handling to AARP-AD, PO Box 51040, Washington, DC 20091.

Making Medical Decisions: Questions and Answers About Health Care Powers of Attorney and Living Wills (D15525) answers often-asked questions to help individuals sort out their values and preferences for end-of-life treatments. AARP, 601 E. St. NW, Washington, DC 20049. No charge.

Planning for Incapacity: A Self-Help Guide to Advance Directives is a state-specific guide containing (1) living will and health-care power-of-attorney forms that comply with the state's laws and practices; (2) easy-to-follow instructions on preparing and individualizing the forms; (3) sensitive discussion of common concerns about advance directives. Indicate your state, send $5 check or money order to LCE, Inc., PO Box 96474, Washington, DC 20090-6474. DC and Virginia residents add applicable sales tax.

Breastfeeding

- *La Leche League* (1-800-LA LECHE), or consult the white pages of the phone book.

- *Breastfeeding Help Line* (sponsored by La Leche League International). (1-900-448-7475) Twenty-four hours a day, seven days a week. Recorded information providing answers to some of the more common problems regarding breastfeeding. As with all

900 numbers there is a charge for this call. The amount of the charge will be given at the beginning of the recording.

- *The Breastfeeding Answer Book*, available from La Leche International.

- *The Womanly Art of Breastfeeding*, La Leche League International, 1991.

Childbirth

- *The Birth Book*, William Sears, MD and Martha Sears, RN. Little, Brown and Company, 1994.

- *A Good Birth, A Safe Birth*, Diana Korte and Roberta Scaer. The Harvard Common Press, 1992.

Children and Hospitals

- *Going To The Hospital*, Fred Rogers. Putnam Sons, 1988.

- *The Berenstain Bears Go To The Hospital*, Stan Berenstain, Random House, New York. 1981. Also comes as a kit with a sound recording. Random House, New York. 1985.

- *Stitches*, Harriet Ziefert. Puffin Books-Penguin.

- *A Visit To The Sesame Street Hospital*, Random House, N.Y.

Relaxation Techniques and Mental Health

- *Prepare for Surgery: Heal Faster*, Peggy Huddleston. Angel River Press.

- *Successful Surgery and Recovery*, Emmett Miller. (audio) Source Cassette Learning Systems. 1980. Distributed by Newman Communications Corp., Albuquerque, N.M.

- *Time Out From Stress*, Matthew McHay, Ph.D. and Patrick Fanning. (audio) New Harbinger Publications, Inc. 5674 Shattuck Ave., Oakland, CA 94609. 1993 Vol. 1 and 2.

- *Ten Minutes To Relax.* (audio) New Harbinger Publications, Inc.

Wellness

- *500 Tips for Coping With A Chronic Illness*, Pamela Jacobs. Robert Reed, Publishers, 1995.

- *Dr. Dean Ornish's Program for Reversing Heart Disease*, Dean Ornish. 1990.

Support Groups

- *American Self-Help Clearinghouse.* 1,000 different selfhelp groups on the Internet. Support and information for people suffering from chronic diseases. Internet address is http://www.cmhc.com/selfhelp/.

NOTES

NOTES

NOTES

NOTES